DEPRESSION

Dealing With Anxiety and Depression With Yoga Poses

(How to Overcome Anxiety, Depression and Change Your Life Forever)

Miranda Sherman

Published By Oliver Leish

Miranda Sherman

All Rights Reserved

Depression: Dealing With Anxiety and Depression With Yoga Poses (How to Overcome Anxiety, Depression and Change Your Life Forever)

ISBN 978-1-77485-257-6

All rights reserved. No part of this guide may be reproduced in any form without permission in writing from the publisher except in the case of brief quotations embodied in critical articles or reviews.

Legal & Disclaimer

The information contained in this book is not designed to replace or take the place of any form of medicine or professional medical advice. The information in this book has been provided for educational and entertainment purposes only.

The information contained in this book has been compiled from sources deemed reliable, and it is accurate to the best of the Author's knowledge; however, the Author cannot guarantee its accuracy and validity and cannot be held liable for any errors or omissions. Changes are periodically made to this book. You must consult your doctor or get professional medical advice before using any of the suggested remedies, techniques, or information in this book.

Upon using the information contained in this book, you agree to hold harmless the Author from and against any damages, costs, and expenses, including any legal fees potentially resulting from the application of any of the information provided by this guide. This disclaimer applies to any damages or injury caused by the use and application, whether directly or indirectly, of any advice or information presented, whether for breach of contract, tort, negligence, personal injury, criminal intent, or under any other cause of action.

You agree to accept all risks of using the information presented inside this book. You need to consult a professional medical practitioner in order to ensure you are both able and healthy enough to participate in this program.

TABLE OF CONTENTS

INTRODUCTION 1

CHAPTER 1: SEARCHING FOR HAPPINESS 2

CHAPTER 2: THE METHOD THROUGH TREATMENTS AND LIFESTYLE CHANGES TO HELP YOU BEAT DEPRESSION 7

CHAPTER 3: TO TREAT DEPRESSION 19

CHAPTER 4: DESIGNING YOUR MAP 31

CHAPTER 5: KEEP ENGAGED 43

CHAPTER 6: ARE YOU JUST EXHAUSTED? 48

CHAPTER 7: THE MOST DEVASTATING THE DISEASE OF MODERN SOCIETY 53

CHAPTER 8: SUPPLEMENTS FOR ANXIETY AND DEPRESSION 69

CHAPTER 9: IN WHAT WAYS DO ALL OF THESE ISSUES AFFECT THIS GENERATION? 77

CHAPTER 10: TREATMENT OPTIONS FOR DEPRESSION 90

CHAPTER 11: WHAT DIFFERENT TYPES OF DEPRESSION?. 94

CHAPTER 12: HOW TO TREAT DEPRESSION? 99

CHAPTER 13: GOAL SETTING YOURSELF GOALS 113

CHAPTER 14: EVIDENCE OF DEPRESSION 118

CHAPTER 15: THE WAY TO BEAT DEPRESSION IN 8 STEPS 130

CHAPTER 16: LIVING WITH DEPRESSION......................... 144

CHAPTER 17: HOW CAN YOU DO? DO ABOUT IT?.......... 153

**CHAPTER 18: THE WAY TO CULTIVATE A POSITIVE
ATTITUDE EVEN WHEN YOU'RE DEPRESSED 167**

CONCLUSION... 180

Introduction

This book provides the most effective steps and strategies on how to conquer depression (and avoid getting back into it) throughout the course the rest of your existence. It provides with all the information you require to remain mentally strong and happy throughout the rest of your life!

I'm sure you're going through some of the most difficult times you've had to go through in your lifetime I'm aware of this because I've been through it myself. I'd like to begin by offering you my deepest gratitude and appreciation for continuing to fight. Things will improve I'm telling you. I am sure of it since you've begun to read this novel. This is a testament to the fact that you'll succeed in this. You are not giving up, and you've not let this defeat you. Together we'll come out the other side and you'll be the better for it.

Chapter 1: Searching For Happiness

There is no one universal definition to happiness. Its significance is determined by the individual whom it is defined by. Whatever the way it's interpreted however, it's still seen as a fundamental human desire. Everyone wants to be happy and content, for if they don't then what's to the point of doing anything? Every decision and action made is designed to satisfy this basic human need.

What is happiness? If you want to give the solution to this question, it is beneficial for us to breakdown it into these concepts:

Happiness is an option. It's incredible that only a tiny portion in happiness -- roughly 10% -- can be attributed to external causes. Actually, a lot of it is the result of our thoughts and experience, rather than the material things we do. This shows that you are in complete control over your feelings and that events don't happen out of luck. If you decide to be satisfied that is, that is what you'll be. If you decide to be depressed and sad If you choose to feel depressed and gloomy, then you'll be. The secret lies in the capacity to manage your feelings. In this regard, it is entirely possible to influence your mind to be content even if you're on the verge of anger. Actually, you could effortlessly let one emotion take over other emotions at whenever you like.

Happiness can be found in many varieties. Everyone has a list of requirements that we are able to keep in mind in the process of determining the things that make us happy or not. Most people's happiness is the result that is based on financial security. If they are able to pay for their luxury items and indulgences, they are content. For some, happiness is from maintaining healthy relationships with family members or friends. They are content with knowing of enhanced by the relationships they decide to maintain. For others they experience happiness from the satisfaction that comes from a positive view of oneself.

Happiness isn't an obscure abstract notion. The chances of you being happy and content could be obscured by your idealized concepts of what happiness actually is. But, it's not helpful to focus on definitions. The most important factor is whether you can put into words the smallest details that make up your life.

Your happiness is what you feel. If, for instance seeking happiness at work, thinking about it in abstract and vague concepts will not bring you anything. Instead, you should opt to focus on the particulars of what you're seeking. Are you working with reliable and trustworthy coworkers? Do you have enough time to travel between the home you live in and workplace just right to stop your from becoming angry? Are the offices at a level that allows you to stay focussed on your work? The answers to these and similar questions will allow you to determine your place at work, and will ultimately provide you with an idea of whether you're truly happy with where you are.

Happiness is an individual and social venture. It is a fact that happiness is something that you need to determine for your own. There is no doubt that you have your own personal criteria to measure happiness, however it's important to remember that the concept of being content extends beyond the self. There is actually an element of social. Your interactions with other people or the way you maintain your relationships with those around you make a significant distinction between being content and content. In the company of those who continually dwell in the negative, for example could affect your ability to see things from a positive perspective and, consequently, influence your perception of happiness.

The best qualities of happiness are revealed individuals. If you're happy you're less likely to be critical of yourself or others' shortcomings. When you focus on the good things that you are happy about, you build a healthy attitude towards yourself and other people. It allows you to become more mature and grow free of limitations and fear that is not substantiated.

Happiness is possible. The most common misconception regarding happiness, is it's something that is a denial of a variety of things that can be achieved including huge homes, money and luxury vehicles, expensive things, and even other tangible wealth. Although it is true that the material wealth may provide a degree of satisfaction for a specific amount of time, this feeling fades when the excitement of the moment disappears and replaced by predictable.

In fact, the secret to happiness is the power of your body and mind be satisfied with the things you control completely. Like we said earlier it is a decision that you make for yourself and it is something that is certainly achievable by a positive attitude and mental outlook.

Chapter 2: The Method Through Treatments and Lifestyle Changes to help you beat depression.

After you've acknowledged your own reality that you actually suffer from depression The next step to consider is finding ways to ease the sadness. There are three avenues you could take in your quest to cure your depression. These are treatment, medication and lifestyle adjustments.

Lifestyle Changes

If the idea of taking drugs or conversing with someone sitting on a couch does not seem appealing to you, it is possible to modify your lifestyle.

Exercise Go out and get active!

Get your sneakers and neon spandex, dance equipment or your attractive swimsuit, and get active. A mere 20-30 minutes each day could result in a dramatic improvement in your mood. It is because exercise increases the serotonin levels, and also releases endorphins. Like antidepressants, exercise stimulates the growth of brain cells. Exercise is a quick and affordable way to test and get rid of the stress. Make sure to vary your routine so that monotony doesn't arise. The worst thing you could do is for your workout that is designed to keep you feeling good, but turns into one that is tedious and you hate. Therefore, go for a walk along gorgeous mountain trails on a beautiful Saturday, do laps of swimming on Tuesdays and then go for a run on Thursday. Take it all in and enjoy yourself.

Change in diet Stop eating sugar.

Diet is as crucial as exercise in relation to your mood. The food you put into your body can impact the overall mood of your mind.

Don't be a snitch!

Below is a list of food items that can cause depression and hindering the improvement of your mood. The foods you should keep out of include:

Refined sugar: Eating sweet foods is certain to bring you happiness for a time as you enjoy that sugary rush. But, it won't last long as that inevitable crash of sugar comes at you like a swarm of bricks. It can make you feel tired and sluggish.

Artificial Sweeteners: Stay clear of drinks and foods that are laced with artificial sweeteners since they can be a cause of depression.

Alcohol: Alcoholic drinks function as depressants. This means that an icy cold glasses of beer could cause an imbalance in the chemical levels within your brain. A regular drinking habit, particularly the consumption of alcohol in excess can eventually lower the serotonin levels in your body, which are the chemical that controls your mood. that is responsible for your mood. Drinking alcohol can also cause stress and anxiety. Additionally, drinking alcohol creates an endless cycle with regards to mood. One drinks alcohol to feel relaxed and happy. calm, however, drinking alcohol can actually lower your mood as time passes. However, many people keep reaching to the bar in search of the feeling of happiness and a opportunity to get rid of sadness. That's an unending cycle. If you're suffering from depression, it's recommended to stay clear of drinking alcohol for an hour.

Caffeine: Research has shown that those who consume excessive amounts of caffeine are much more susceptible to depression when as compared to those who don't drink caffeinated drinks. In a world populated by tea and coffee drinkers it's not too over the top to insist on abstaining entirely from caffeine. Therefore, it is recommended to consume caffeinated beverages in moderation. Limit yourself to 2 cup of coffee, or 3-4 cups tea.

Yes, you can eat and drink!

After we've looked at the foods that can make you feel depressed Here's a variety of foods that will help increase your mood. Foods you must consider buying include:

Nuts: Specifically, almonds as well as cashews, walnuts, brazil nuts. Consuming 1-2 brazil nuts per day has been proven to increase the levels of serotonin in an individual's.

Fresh vegetables and fruits The fact is that it has always been well-known that fruits and vegetables are beneficial for your health. They have often been mentioned by books, parents as well as the small pamphlets available at doctors' offices. Your mind is not immune to these advantages. Eating fresh fruit and vegetables can aid in helping to ease depression. Avocado, asparagus blueberries, raspberries, and blackberries are particularly effective to boost your mood.

Chamomile as well as green tea Chamomile tea is best consumed prior to laying down because it helps you sleep more peacefully. This means that you will get an unrestricted sleep that isn't full of anxiety and discomfort. Green tea is many benefits as well as helping to combat depression. Drink 2 glasses of tea each day.

Wholegrain bread

Cottage cheese

Oatmeal

Brain Food: Consume plenty of food that contain omega-3, since this essential fatty acid may help boost your mood. Most seafood and olive oil are particularly abundant in this essential fatty acid.

Sleep in Take advantage of your sleep

It's not exactly fun to get to bed at the normal time of 10:30-11pm, however 7 to 8 hours of sleep per night could have a major effect upon your mental state. If you are up all night with your eyes glued to the computer (I'm looking at the tumbler in front of you], you're more likely to be irritable and cranky, as well as in the larger picture, it could make your depression worse. The hours of restful and peaceful sleep are crucial in your strategy to beat depression off its grim backside.

Yoga

30-40 minutes of exercise every day, is very beneficial to your mood as well as your overall health. Yoga is beneficial because it reduces anxiety and stress. It provides you with a period of time throughout the day when you'll be in a state of relaxation. It also assists in lifting your mood and increasing self-esteem through building the body and shaping it. Serotonin levels are also increased through regularly practiced yoga.

Counselling or Therapy

This type of treatment could be administered alongside medication or alone and involves addressing issues or issues that make you feel uneasy. The first thing you need to consider regarding this type of treatment is whom you'll be talking to. For this, first ask a family member or your physician for the names of counselors or therapists who are recommended. Then, schedule appointments with the names that appear at the top of the list. Visit them and see what you think about them. Does it make you feel at ease? Perhaps the reverse is true are they making you feel uncomfortable and uncomfortable? Additionally, consider the room where the therapy is taking place. Are they warm and cozy or cold and sterile? Find a location and a the person who creates the most hospitable environment. If that means getting to know various people until you can find the right one, that's fine. It's about you and your efforts to get rid of the debilitating sadness that you've been entrapped in.

Therapy is beneficial for helping to reduce depression due to a variety of reasons. It can be extremely therapeutic to talk about things in your life which have brought anxiety or grief for example, divorce or the death of the family. Therapy can also help you develop ways to manage depression, as well as attempting to alter your thinking or behaviors, such as becoming less self-critical of yourself.

Medication

If you choose to go to a doctor to help you with depression, they may suggest using antidepressants. Antidepressants may be prescribed to help relieve symptoms of clinical depression and the seasonal affective disorder (SAD) and dysthymia. There are many kinds of antidepressants on the market that help in relieving depression-related symptoms. The most commonly used type of medication prescribed is selective serotonin reuptake inhibitors , or SSRIs. They function by increasing the levels of serotonin as well as noradrenaline which are two substances found within the brain that affect mood. The typical classes of antidepressants that are available to patients these in the present include Citalopram, Paroxetine, Zoloft, Lexapro, Prozac, Cymbalta, Venlafaxine and Luvox.

It is vital to keep in mind that there are certain negative side effects people can suffer from while taking antidepressants. These include:

Nausea

Fatigue

Incapacity to create

An absence of desire for sexual activity

A higher level of anxiety

Unrest

Dizziness

Gain in weight

Dry mouth

Changes in the bowel movement

Headaches

Extreme sweating

Suicidal thoughts are increasing

Many adverse side-effects will diminish within the initial three weeks of taking anti-depressants.

Antidepressants aren't an addiction drug, however, there are risks when you abruptly cease using these medications. If you want to stop using this kind of drug you must talk to a doctor. They will devise an appropriate plan to gradually and gradually reduce your use of the medication so that no negative side effects occur. If you abruptly stop taking antidepressants , a variety of negative side effects may be experienced. These being:

Nausea

Headaches

Anxiety

Vomiting

Extreme mood shifts

Insomnia

Quick to rise up to anger

Dizziness

Lack of coordination

Brain shocks: a strange sensation that feels as that your brain is shocked.

Sometimes, these shocks can be experienced in other areas of the body.

The shakes

In the case of psychosis depression alternative treatment approach is required , which is hospitalization. In hospital the patient is provided with the adequate care and support, along with medications in the form of antidepressants and antipsychotic drugs that aid in stopping hallucinations.

Chapter 3: To Treat Depression

If people are thinking of treatments and cures for medical conditions such as depression, they typically consider hospitalization and medication. They usually focus on the methods of science, but they don't be aware of the alternatives that are natural and available. Natural methods can be as effective as their medical counterparts. Note that they've been around longer and people have used them for centuries.

If you suffer from depression, you must be aware that taking medication could be more risky and harmful as compared to natural methods of treatment. Apart from the potential loss of these drugs they can also cause various unpleasant negative side consequences. If you don't want to risk it You can opt for alternative treatments that are natural, such as the following:

Physical or Movement

The body's exercise triggers it to release endorphins. These are natural chemicals that work with the receptors in your brain. They work as an alkaline or painkiller that stimulate positive feelings that your body produces. They are similar like the opioid morphine.

According to a research study published within the Journal of Sport and Exercise Psychology exercise can increase endorphin levels as well as pump the heart. This can boost your mood and help alleviate depression. The Dr. David Muzina, director of the Cleveland Clinic Center for Mood Disorders Treatment and Research, stated that exercise can trigger the release of brain-related chemicals if you suffer from depression. Some of the simple but efficient exercises you can perform include yoga, running strengthening exercises, walking at a fast pace.

Diet

A balanced and healthy diet can help you fight depression. Be aware that the food you eat directly impacts your thinking and behave. Researchers have discovered that a bad diets can cause the development of depression. A poor diet is typically comprised of sugars, fried food, fried foods unhealthy fats, dairy products, refined grains along with processed animal products.

If you are looking to beat depression naturally, you must to ensure that you are eating a diet rich in antioxidants to fight free radicals and damaging molecules that can cause ageing, cell damage and dysfunction. The best sources of antioxidants are fruits, apricots and carrots and collars, spinach, sweet potato, berries seeds, nuts and cantaloupes.

Another approach to easing depression is to remain at peace with a healthy and balanced diet. You can reap the soothing effects of carbs like legumes as well as fruits and vegetables. Be sure to take omega-3 fatty acids from mackerel, tuna and salmon, sardines, as well as other fish with fatty content. Doctors and nutritionists also suggest drinking green tea since it helps reduce the symptoms and signs of depression.

Supplements

It's a fact that you should keep a healthy lifestyle to avoid diseases. Sometimes it is the case that a healthy diet isn't enough. This is the reason you might require supplements to ensure that your body is getting the nutrition it needs.

Vitamin D such as helps enhance bone health and mental well-being. According to research, vitamin D receptors are located in various areas within the brain. They are situated on the cells' surface which receive chemical signals which instruct cells to take the required action. Note that some of your brain's receptors are in turn vitamin D receptors meaning vitamin D works in a unique way within your brain.

They are located in brain areas which are linked to depression. Therefore vitamin D may also be associated with depression as well as other mental health issues. It may affect the quantity of monoamines, like serotonin and how they function in the brain. Antidepressants are used to increase the monoamine content that are present in brain. Vitamin D works the same way. It also boosts the level of monoamines that are present in the brain, and aids in fighting against depression.

Brain Dump Journaling

Journaling is frequently suggested to people suffering from depression due to it being an effective and relaxing method to share emotions and thoughts in a relaxed and unprejudiced manner, without having to worry about hurting other people or being thought of as a victim. If you write your thoughts in your journal, you're the only person who can read your thoughts written on paper. Therefore, you won't be embarrassed or shy. You can speak as much as you want to without fear of repercussions which allows you to pour out all of your unresolved feelings.

Journaling allows you to connect with areas of your mind which have been secluded. Journaling also lets you draw on the deep reservoirs of problem-solving and imagination. When you write in a journal you experience a flash of awareness and a sense of knowing that you've never experienced before.

As per Dr. Michael Rank, co-director and associate professor at the International Traumatology Institute of the University of South Florida, journaling can force journal keepers perform something. In the words of Dr. Jessie Gruman, executive director of the Center for the Advancement of Health in Washington believes that journaling is a fantastic method to deal with depression. Journaling also provides you with an chance to look at your emotions written in black and white which gives you time to work out the best ways to manage them.

Breathing Exercises

Breathing becomes slow when you feel stressed or feeling low. This is not a great indicator because breathing shallowly could cause emotional instability. This can reduce the oxygen in blood. However, this issue is easily solved with deep breathing and acupressure.

Through acupuncture, acupuncture points that are potent are applied to the skin. This increases blood circulation. When you breathe deeply, huge amounts of air are absorbed while exhaling slowly. This increases the benefits of acupressure , as and increases the supply of oxygen. When you breathe deeply and maintain a steady rhythm you will increase the amount of oxygen that is delivered to your lungs, blood and organs, as well as cells. Remember that oxygen is essential to maintaining the functioning of your body's physiological systems. Breathing deeply relaxes your body and mind and helps change negative thoughts into positive ones.

Cold/Hot Therapy

The temperature can impact a range of things, not just the way you feel. This is the reason why the use of hot and cold therapies is utilized to reduce depression. Experts have also devised the idea of a hot tent in order to combat depression. A person suffering from depression is put in the tent, and then pulls out his head while the body is still in the. The temperature in the tent increases the body's temperature, that triggers the release of chemical substances in the brain.

Cold therapy operates in similarly, causing similar physiological stressors to the primates that they have endured throughout their evolution. It's been proven that lack of heat exercise can hinder the brain's functioning. If you suffer from depression, you should consider treatment with cold water. Your body will be exposed to the frigid temperature of the water flowing, which causes your brain and body to experience a physiological reaction. Researchers from Virginia Commonwealth University School of

Medicine Virginia Commonwealth University School of Medicine have discovered that patients suffering from depression who received cold showers have seen significant improvements in their mood.

Change Who You Hang Out With (End toxic relationships)

According to researchers at The University of Warwick and the University of Manchester, maintaining an active social network can ease stress and help to prevent the development of depression. The World Health Organization (WHO) reporting over 350 million people who suffer from depression, the subject of depression is now an issue of great issue.

The research team has discovered that the most important factor in determining the best ways to treat and prevent depression is becoming aware of the social factors that trigger and cause it. If you're trying to be happier, you need pick your employer carefully. You must surround yourself with positive and positive people to absorb their positive vibes. Positive moods can be spread more easily due to the notion of imitation amongst your friends.

Support Groups

People who are depressed frequently request to be by themselves. They prefer to lock themselves in their bedrooms and are unable to interact with people. But, this approach isn't beneficial. If you suffer from depression and feel as if you're being in a lonely place, you need to take a break and find an aid group. If you are surrounded by people around you, you are able to clear your worry away. If you're with friends who understand exactly what you're going through You can feel calm.

A support group much better than talking to a family or friend member, because members of the group understand what you are feeling and what are experiencing. They are also depressed and you don't have to justify yourself every time. The people who do not suffer from depression might not be able to comprehend how it feels to be afflicted with an illness like yours. If you're part of your group of support and you are able to be you without fear about being assessed.

Additionally, you'll be able to take advantage of their advice and suggestions as and listen to their personal struggles, stories, etc. Their experiences can inspire and motivate you. Also, you can gain important lessons from their stories. If you are unable to locate an organization that is close to your location, you may sign up to an online group.

Self-Help and alternative therapies

Patients suffering from depression may also ameliorate their symptoms through lifestyle modifications and other solutions like the following:

Meditation

Meditation is widely known to enhance the condition of mind and body. Anyone suffering from depression can manage their emotions and thoughts by practicing meditation.

Aromatherapy

Massage or inhaling essential oils onto your body may have soothing and relaxation effects. Essential oils contain soothing and therapeutic properties that can assist you to manage depression.

Acupuncture

It is the process of using extremely fine needles which stimulate specific parts in the human body. It helps you relax and soothe your mind and also assist you in fighting depression.

Herbal remedies

A large number of people seek out natural remedies to find alternatives to prescription medications. St. John's wort is one of the most well-known natural remedy to treat depression. It may help improve mood levels.

Chapter 4: Designing Your Map

What you must create is a set of routines that will get you to the desired place. I'll teach you how to make costumes that will help you develop your own habits!

It is the first step to trace yourself. Find out where you are now and where you'd like to be. We can do this by recognizing the habits you're currently using. Here's how to do it. On a piece of paper, write:

1. Write what you are feeling. Write about your feelings if you're feeling depressed, lonely, sad, angry or anxious or whatever other emotion you believe you're experiencing. Make sure you're specific!

2. Write down your list of your daily routines. These are the actions you perform to bring you closer to your emotions. Make sure you are specific! There are many rituals that you can do during the day that help you to be being the way you are. If you consider them and then write them down, you'll be able to identify them and become self-aware.

Make sure you are thorough beginning from the moment you wake up until the time you go to bed and you are in bed. Be sure to think about it and be precise!

Consider as many practices you practice every day that lead to your goal. Write down all the things you do throughout the day, the way you think about during the day, and also your facial expression and posture throughout the day.

These are some common questions to assist you. Answer the followingquestions:

Your Mind

What should I be focusing on? The good or the negative that I am experiencing in life? What should I be focusing on particularly?

Do I get caught up in an unfortunate or a difficult situation? Do I dwell on one or a few? Note them down.

Do I engage in positive or negative self-talk? What do I really say?

Your Physiology

What should I do with my body physiology when I'm depressed?

Do I need to cry?

Do I slump?

Do I smile or look down?

Are I cranky?

Your Personal Habits

Do you indulge in fast food that isn't nutritious, skip meals or overindulge?

Do you find yourself in front of a computer or sitting at your desk looking at your computer unproductively?

Do I sit idle or do I exercise? How long can I sit at a desk or work out?

3. Write what you want to write. This is the destination you've always wanted to reach. In the event that you could have unlimited money the world, how would wish to live your life every day? Make it clear!

Unlimited resources refers to the fact that money was not an issue, nor your health, or your relationships or relationships, etc.

Live life to the fullest, that is what would you like to feel and feel the world as you live it. Don't be a slave to materialistic desires, but real life experiences. Make sure you are specific!

Think about a typical Tuesday when your kids go to school , and you head to work. What's the ideal way to "love" for a Tuesday? There are no parties or other crazy things that could cause you to die even if you were to do them everyday. A normal day type of things and in a manner that you'd love to go through.

Imagine your entire day, beginning with waking up in your bed, going about your usual daily routine and then getting back to the bed and falling to sleep. What do you want your day to be? Make sure you are specific!

Let's look at an instance:

"I would like to get up and smile easily, feel refreshed, and know that the new dawn is shining beautifully and brightly over me, full of possibilities and joy."

"I am up and put on my shoes and head for a pleasant, energetic walk. I then go for go for a run in a stunning setting, brimming in gratitude while feeling the energy and strength of exercising my body and reviving my mind"

"I am looking forward to sharing my playtime with my husband and have fun with the silly and fun things my kids play with."

"I wish to feel the joy and joy of having accomplished something exceptional at work and be confident that I've done excellent work at what I do."

"I would like to make friends for lunch with my partner and eat healthy food and engage in meaningful, interesting and engaging conversations."

"I am hoping to take my kids from school and spend some time to play outdoors with them, playing with them in their fun games, and cherishing their innocent innocence."

"I enjoy a full healthy, delicious, and nutritious dinner with my family and we discuss our day's activities and we smile a bit when we share stories."

"I get ready for bed, and pull out a book to read for an hour or so, being in a quiet space with my husband at my side."

"I am able to sleep in a serene and clean bedroom, happy and exhausted, and confident that I've contributed to my family as well as my friends and society and thankful that I was given an opportunity to give it."

"I sleep tired, but content and peaceful."

Be as precise that you are able to. Include as much as you are able to. Every day, if your mind can manage it. The more detailed you can get into, the better it will be to be able to live it out in your mind.

Extend your imagination and force to think of the most memorable moments you can ever experience. It's for as long as you'd like. The sky is the limit!

You're doing great! Keep working. Then, write the next.

4. What are the daily habits I "Should" do to achieve the experiences I want. It's not easy to implement them however if you were able to follow the routines that you're accustomed to when life is perfect simply write them down. Make sure you are precise!

If you had a life that was wonderful and beautiful, write about it. Include your body's posture and facial expressions frequently.

Make sure you are specific about what rituals and routines you perform every day to lead to the desired life experience. The posture of the body and facial expression are crucial. Remember that the mind and body are inextricably linked.

These are some possible questions that can aid you in your answer:

What do I consider when I wake up? Do I smile and think of things that I'm thankful for?

What can I do about my posture, body and facial posture throughout my day? Stand up and sit straight? Keep looking up? Concentrate on the gorgeous sky frequently?

Do I exercise? What type of exercise do I prefer? What would I like to do when I exercise? Was there a sport from my childhood that I loved to play? What was the duration? How often ? precisely do I train?

What can me do, and what am I thinking about at breakfast?

What do I do and what do I talk over with my parents?

What is my body's face and posture?

What should I think and do when I get to work? How should I conduct myself, how do I interact with my colleagues during the course of my day?

What can I do to have lunch?

What is my body's facial expression and posture?

What should you do? What do I think of after work, when I get to bed?

What should I do once I return back

What can I do to prepare at dinner, and what should I say to my family?

What is my body's face and posture?

What can I do to prepare myself for ending my day and going to sleep?

If you require help with your list look over the next chapter to learn positive actions you can accomplish.

5. Write down your Desired Habit Liste of Desired Habits. Make a list of your desirable habits, put it in a place where you will view it each day like your mirror or bathroom wall and practice these habits every day for 30 consecutive days.

Create a copy of the document and place it in your workplace!

If you fall off in one day, retake for the next 30 days. Habits are hard to break if they're not used, so continue making the activities you have listed until they become routine and replace your previous routines.

The circumstances of your life aren't changing. Your marriage might remain a mess or the loved one, who might have passed away, but will not return, as well as numerous other external factors. However, you've got a list of aspects "You" can accomplish and manage.

Your life will be influenced by positive thoughts. It's essential in your life to be attracted to the things you believe. Keep making lists and practice it.

Try these. Test them. Have fun with it. Add it to your list and record it so that you can look back and try it out.

You've been practicing for a long time in order to be the depressed person. Why not just pretend and try the new method? What's the worst thing that could occur? You may still stay depressed. Therefore, you've not lost anything.

If you follow the steps you have written in your checklist, I'll guarantee you a life-changing experience!

You'll notice that the little things that alter. One thing at a. Have you ever felt deja vu before? Have you ever thought about someone who you hadn't seen for an extended period of time, only to encounter the person in a surprising manner?

The power behind attraction is. Everyone has this power. With enough effort we can attract whatever we can imagine. If you repeat it enough then you'll become an habit.

Habits are only formed when you do them for thirty days in a row. If you fall short on the rules, simply restart the calendar and continue for a further 30 days.

This is known as the Law of Attraction. It's true. It's been discussed on television and the movie "The secret."

Once you have mastered how to attract people, I'll give you the specific behaviors to adopt that will help you transition from despair to joy.

Chapter 5: Keep Engaged

Let's look at another issue that is common among depressed people the depressed: overthinking.

In general, and we are given the chance we can think on a subject for quite a long period of time. This is normal and very beneficial in certain instances: it could assist you in determining what was wrong with a particular situation and determine the corrective actions to take.

The problem comes when this thought process is stretched over a particular threshold, particularly when the thought process is based on negative thoughts.

It's as simple as:

After a while of thinking about what was not working, you will be able to think of all kinds of solutions that can improve the situation which is a positive thing.

In the next few days, you'll hit a limit of your returns, when any further thought turns into little or no insight into the subject. In that case it is best in getting out of the rut and focusing your energy to something different.

Most individuals, one of the issue is that we could endure this pattern for many hours, creating making depression a recipe.

Here's the reason:

The way that overthinking can lead to depression

The brain's stress response mechanism or the fight or flight response. This mechanism will be activated no matter if the scenario is real or imaginary. However, the majority times our negative thoughts are misguided conclusion about a situation that could be perceived as threatening.

People who are depressed tend to do this until it becomes second-nature. Therefore, it is difficult for a person suffering from depression to break a negative chain of thoughts. However, there is an opportunity.

Hope is in the simple fact obsessional thoughts only take root when you've got nothing else to do.

For example consider the time you are idle in your daily life, such as during traffic jams or eating, taking a break after work and so on. It is interesting that your free period is when you're most likely to be susceptible to negative thoughts patterns.

Being busy is among the most effective ways to avoid negative thoughts.

Do something that is physically and mentally challenging that will distract you from your thoughts that are negative. If you do this, you'll be so absorbed in the work you do that you barely notice the passing of time.

What is the reason that doing things that are physically and mentally demanding aid in reducing depression? It's because it's impossible to concentrate on several things simultaneously at a single time. The human brain doesn't possess that capacity!

It is possible to only concentrate only one thing at a given time and can't think about two things at once. Do it. Think about someone you can picture in your head-- perhaps your mother. And think about the dinner you'll cook later on in the day. It's difficult to concentrate on two things at once. That's the power of meditation.

The inability of our minds to concentrate upon two different things at time is among the numerous reasons that occupational therapy is a powerful treatment for depression. Therapists with a specialization in this area of expertise suggest "work" on their patients in order to help them deal with anxiety, depression as well as other psychological disorders. This treatment has been in use for a long time.

This method works for me. If I'm stressed about something, then I know I'll probably fall into depression. So, I put my mind's energy in doing something constructive. I do some work--you know, such as writing the book you're currently reading.

In the end I'm immersed in work, to the point that I don't think about my problems. The time passes by in such a speed that I barely remember that the day is done. As soon as it's bedtime I fall asleep then call it an night.

The majority of people are negative toward work. Work is truly a blessing. It can take the mind off of your anxieties and enable you to achieve many things in your life, which means you get the most out of both things.

Being worried about the things that make depression more likely will do exactly the opposite. It's not going to accomplish anything when you're anxious and depressed, and it will make your life more difficult.

Steps to take

I encourage you to adopt the concept of working as a treatment for depression and observe how it affects your life to the positive.

Chapter 6: Are You Just Exhausted?

In the first chapter , we discovered that depression can be an indication from our feelings that is the an appropriate time to slow down and breathe or take a break and think about the direction we're moving towards, or maybe be faced with things that are very challenging for us.

There could be a different reason to your depressive mood that is not specific messages that come from our thoughts or external life situations. It could be that you are tired of your mind.

Another aspect of modern western society is that we're constantly being bombarded by information and demands for our attention and energy. Our jobs are less physically demanding but more draining mentally. Our working days pass through in a blur of continuous thinking, problem-solving and multi-tasking. We might have the time to unwind from this constant thinking , by relaxing on the couch or watching another form of entertainment, or even a narcotic that is that is designed to temporarily force our minds off.

But, these strategies do not work well. Do this for a test. Take a break from reading, shut your eyes and observe how long before your mind begins to whirl around, thinking about the other and this, worry and imagining things as well as bouncing around and generally making a mess.

The constant activity of our minds becomes extremely exhausting quickly. It's not the same as physical exhaustion. It may (after an intense exercise session for instance) actually feel extremely pleasant. It's just an ache, a feeling of numbness or feeling disconnected from the world that is very often a sign of depression.

How can we stop this? The answer is in the ancient and now extensively researched area of meditation. Meditation gives us the chance to relax our tired mind and then to recharge it until you feel refreshed as well as relaxed, energized and rejuvenated.

The following exercise is an intro to the practice of meditation. I suggest doing this in a secure in a quiet, peaceful and comfortable space in which you aren't interrupted for a minimum of 10 minutes.

1. Remain in a straight and still position, say to you that over the next 10 minutes (or the time you decide to set) you'll just observe your breathing and relax . whatever else comes to your mind , you'll let it go to be aware of it and observe.

2. Begin to observe your breathing. This is simply refer to paying close attention to how you breath. Your mind may wander. If this happens you can forgive yourself and bring the focus back on your breathing. If you find yourself thinking about something else, just watch the situation, and get back to breathing.

3. There are three parts of your breathing that you should be watching. The first one is the inhalation. The second is exhalation. The third part is the small intervals between breathing in and out. For a short

time the breath ceases. It is an significant moment to observe because your mind will be at peace in the moment.

4. There are three essential components to meditation. The first is awareness. Be attentive to what happens. Stay conscious. Be conscious. The second state is one of relaxation. Do not strain, do not worry simply relax. The more you relax the more comfortable do not push any thing. Thirdly, non-judgment. whatever comes to your mind Don't make judgments about it as bad or good positive or negative Just observe it and return to your breathing when you're at your best.

5. Once your time has expired take a moment to slowly close your eyes and go through your day. The longer and more deeply you are meditative the more relaxed and rejuvenated you'll feel.

Meditation can be a wonderful remedy to our modern way of living and the stress of our jobs. Make the effort to practice this. It's not a bad idea! Most people come out of meditation with a sense of tranquility, healing and peace. Meditation can be performed at any time , and feel at ease to spend whatever time you like during each session. It can transform your entire life!

Chapter 7: The Most Devastating

The Disease Of Modern Society

How can depression be defined?

Does it have to be a condition?

Does it stem from a brain malfunction which can be corrected?

Are there biochemical imbalances?

Is it a present problem that arises as an outcome of our style of life?

Is this a global issue that it is described by the World Health Organization mentions?

What's the story behind this disease that is sweeping into our lives, and its effects alter our balance in our families or our personal lives?

On 10thOctober 2012 10th October 2012, World Mental Health Day was focused on depression and its impact on our lives. It is reported that the World Health Organization mentions that around the world, over 350 million suffer from depression. Depression is a serious mental illness that is characterised by sadness, demotivation in life, poor concentration, guilt or low self- worth, fatigue and insomnia or food disturbances.

It is a widespread illness and it is important to be aware that it is feasible for everyone to be affected by it. It is also known as "black dog". Winston Churchill, a man with whose fate Britain was entrusted was afflicted by major depressive episodes which he referred to as "black dog". There is little we know of Winston Churchill's "black dog". Many historians refused to acknowledge that leaders could be depressed. It is believed that the most powerful men will not be suffering from mental illness and, if they do, it's better to ignore it and never discuss it.

Even though everyone else was content to ignore his symptoms of depression, Churchill named his illness as "Black Dog" and acknowledged the fact that "... I do not prefer standing on the edge of the platform when an express train is going through. I prefer to stay behind and, if I can create a pillar that is in between myself and my train. I'm not a fan of standing at the end of a ship looking at the ocean. One second of action could end all things. A handful of drops of

desperation..."

In a letter to his doctor he explains his thoughts on depression to his wife "I believe this doctor could help me, should my black dog return. It's not too far from me at present - it is an amazing feeling. All colors return to me". There is no way to avoid the possibility of being depressed However, it appears like this "black dog" has a tendency to stigmatize everyone, with no exceptions.

Some Statistical Information about Depression

The mental illness depression is one condition that is more frequent than other. It is often referred to as the most debilitating disease of the 21st century as it has risen quickly. According to research, one out of ten people be affected by depression at any time in their lives. As far as disabilities, death and social problems depression is ranked as the fourth among the most serious diseases in the world. It is predicted that by 2020, depression will rank first within Western societies.

Research on epidemiology shows that women are affected by depression around the world, more often than males.

The likelihood of having depression during a lifetime ranges from 10% to 20 percent for females, and between 5% and 12% for males. It doesn't matter whether they reside in low or high-income nations, the World Health Organization (2008) declares it is depression that's the most prevalent reason for illness that affects women.

What is the reason women suffer from depression more often than males?

* Biological issues that relate to the etiology behind depression.

* Based on studies of fraternal and identical twins and family historical records, it appears the case that women have a greater genetic predisposition to depression in women than in males.

* Differences in hormones between males and females Women have more

changes in hormone levels are more frequent than men , and this can be linked to depression symptoms.

* Stressful life situations (birth and raising children) that women are exposed, are believed to be the reason for the different the rates of men and women.

Due to their greater involvement in relationships with their families than males and women, they are more vulnerable when relationships are shattered. The responsibilities of family and work are often juggled and challenging to manage. It's frequently for women to look after an elderly family member and also.

* It has been found that women suffering with depressive disorders are much more likely to get assistance and have a greater chance of receiving an earlier diagnosis as well as treatment. Sexual prejudices and psychological factors hinder men from seeking out with a doctor. The men have learned that the expression of negative emotions is a sign of weakness and that men must always be confident. Many young youngsters are being taught the idea that men don't let themselves cry! If they are unhappy, they need to shut down their feelings! Discussing sadness or weak points is considered a "female privilege" therefore men are resisted from seeking assistance. Physicians are more likely to diagnose depression among women, than males. More likely is that male symptoms are related to anxiety disorders, but not depression.

Depression can happen at any time and usually begins at an early age. There is a increasing concern that as much as between 2% and five percent of children might have depression. Children who are more prone to depression may have lost their parents at an early age, having to face issues of abandonment. Poor academic performance, unhealthy social relationships, and addiction to substances are the results of depression in teens and children's lives.

The typical age of depression symptoms starts around the age of 25. The increased consumption of alcohol and other drugs can be linked to depression episodes within the aforementioned age ranges. It is more frequent in adult females and adolescent girls than in adolescent or adult males. There is no distinction in frequency between males as well as females in the time of preadolescence. The highest risk of suffering from depression in both women is between the ages of 25 and 44 years old. The rate of depression decreases by both genders after the age of 65.

Depression disorders tend to be recurrent and affect human function. As compared to other conditions depression is the reason for absenteeism from work and school within the range of 15 to 45. People who suffer from an episode of depression but are not treatedfor it, are more likely to have a 50% chance of having a second episode within the next five years. The probability of recurrence of an episode of depression is 90 percent after three depressive episodes.

Depression sufferers are frequently considered to be a stigmatized group. This means that many individuals aren't aware they are suffering from depression and many do not seek treatment. One in three of those suffering from depression is treated. With the proper treatment depression can be overcome with a success rate of between 80 and 90 percent. Despite the effectiveness of treatment, many people aren't receiving it. Lack in resources and the deficiency of professionals who are trained and skilled and the stigma associated with being diagnosed with a mental illness appear to be the reasons the reason that the majority of people who suffer aren't receiving effective treatment.

Depression is a disorder that more frequently than other illness can cause someone to suicide. People who suffer from depressive episodes that are severe suffer from high suicide rates of up to 15 percent. Every 11/2 minute, a man is killed through suicide, and suicide attempts can be numerous.

According to the World Health Organization (2012) nearly a million lives have been lost to suicide. That means that 3000 people take their own lives every day. Each time somebody attempts suicide, at least 20 could try to end their lives.

Chronic illness is an important factor in creating depression-related symptoms. Anyone suffering from chronic illness are more likely to experience depression. In the end, they are more depressed and their physical condition is severely deteriorated.

Are you depressed or sad?

Some people wonder when it's moment to seek assistance. The earlier treatment is started better it will be. What is the difference between depression and sadness?

Following a loss, divorce or a failure individuals may experience feelings of emotions of sadness, despair, and discontent. When this happens it's not unusual to feel depressed. The feelings are an expression of the grief of loss. These feelings are normal when they do not impact the person's everyday functioning. It is true that being aware of our emotions triggers emotional processing of negative events and it assists us in getting out of these challenging situations.

Clinical depression is distinct from feelings of sadness and fatigue. The main thing that distinguishes depression isn't the existence of negative emotions but their intense intensity and persistence that impact people's lives daily. The depressive mood is not affected by the environment the person is in. For instance, they won't be happy or smile at the midst of a happy event. The depressive mood can be the most severe in the morning. Even when they do manage to fall asleep, they are aware that they are not able to be peaceful or relaxed.

Unmasking The Truths About Depression

Prejudices and stereotypes that are associated with depression as well as the lack of information are serious for those suffering from depression. Due to stigmatization, many people are hesitant to seek assistance. Dispelling the myths that are associated with depression is a vital step toward removing prejudices and discrimination in the social realm.

The earlier we become informed and know the real cause of this depression quicker we will be able to find ways to aid people who are in need. If we can dispel the myths that confuse us, the quicker we will discover the answers to our questions. The earlier we challenge stereotypes, the faster depression's truth will be revealed. It won't be dark. It will be the truth.

Dispelling the myths surrounding depression helps us be more prepared to fight this illness.

1. Depression is an indicator of weakness.

Patients with depression are viewed as weak, just like people who quit on life. Depression is a complicated mental illness that no one decides to treat. Instructing them to take action or telling them they're not doing enough can make them feel frustrated lonely, depressed and lost. Instead, standing with them without judging their efforts will help to encourage them to seek assistance.

2.Traumatic life situations can lead to depression.

Though life events that are traumatic may trigger depressive episodes, it isn't the norm. Many sufferers may experience depression without having experienced trauma. Traumatic experiences provoke negative feelings. In addition to the severity as well as the duration and frequency are the most important aspects to look for assistance.

3. Depression isn't a real illness.

Depression is a debilitating mental illness that can affect every aspect of life. It's not about character or the persona one is. This is a medical problem that can affect individuals on a physical, emotional and social level.

4. It's everything in your mind.

Try to motivate an acquaintance or loved one by saying it's all in the mind can make them feel less strong. Depression can be a debilitating mental illness with physical manifestations that are severe, like appetite or sleep issues, fatigue, chest pains and muscle aches. The absence of physical symptoms and not thinking about them can be a deterrent of contacting the loved one person suffering from depression.

5.Men and depression aren't a good match together.

According to the literature, men are affected by depression just as often as women. Men's stereotypes of stable, strong and masculine males not speaking up about their emotions and not being open about their concerns cause depression to be more risky for men. In the absence of seeking help, people usually resort to using substances. There is a report that suggests suicides are much more effective for males. What is the reason for this? Men don't just resort to more violent methods to put the end of their lives but also fail to receive the diagnosis.

6.Like father Like son, like father.

It is believed you should know that when your parents suffer from depression, you will too. This is completely false. Although genetic predisposition may increase the chance of developing depression, it's not enough. Individuals who have a family history of depression live in the shadows of their fears of being diagnosed with depression. The only thing the can be done is be aware of their symptoms and seek out help in the event that they really require it.

7.Antidepressants are the only treatment for depression.

The antidepressants they are usually not sufficient. They alter brain chemistry and lessen the severity of depression symptoms. However, is it enough? Through psychotherapy, those suffering from depression are able to recognize the issues in their lives and establish achievable goals. Thoughts that are negative or distorted can be detected through psychotherapy. Psychotherapy helps to restore the sense of control and happiness in your life. It has been found that taking therapy and medication are the most effective approach to managing depression.

8.Talking about thoughts and feelings can make it worse.

If you are able to suppress the negative emotions you are like the eruption of a volcano. It's set to occur. Traumas and negative emotions are not able to heal by themselves. Speaking about your thoughts and feelings won't make the situation worse. It's more of a way to get the help that you require.

Chapter 8: Supplements for Anxiety and Depression

It is crucial to take a few supplements to ease depression and stress. In this section, we'll review some supplements you must consume in order to relieve yourself of these issues as quickly as possible.

Vitamin D

There is a belief that vitamin D deficiency causes producing cortisol within the brain which can cause stress to rise. Therefore, it is essential for you to have an x-ray of your blood to examine the level of vitamin D within your body. If you are deficient, then you must consult your physician to determine the most effective vitamin D supplement to your body. The dosage will vary from person to person , and when you live in an area with limited sunlight, you need to take a greater dosage as compared to those who reside in sunny areas.

Omega 3 fat acids

Omega 3 fats are necessary to ensure good brain function. It is a source of DHA which is essential for brain function and the health of the brain. According to studies by women suffering depressive symptoms, they observed that 30% of them had this chemical at the brains of those with low amounts. It is possible to consume fish oils to combat this issue, since they are extremely high in omega 3 acid fatty acids. You can grind flax seeds, and add them to salads or dissolving in water and drink, as they are extremely high in omega 3 fatty acids.

Rhodiola

Rhodiola is a plant that is utilized to treat mental illnesses. It's believed to assist in reducing stress which could result from physical and environmental stimuli. It is said that you will feel calmer and relaxed when you take this herb , and it can also aid in reducing anxiety and stress. Rhodiola can also be helpful in helping to induce sleep, and you'll notice that your worries are beginning to diminish. It can be purchased in tablet form and can be purchased at online stores.

Gingko

Gingko is a plant which is high in antioxidants and helps in reducing damage from oxidative in the brain. Gingko assists in reducing stress as well as stress associated side consequences. It can also be used to provide relief from headaches and migraine. It assists in boosting circulation of brain blood. You'll feel more energized and full of life after you start taking this herb. It is accessible in tablets and can be taken for immediate release from anxiety.

Lavender

Lavender is a plant that can be used to treat anxiety and stress-related disorders. It is mostly employed to induce restful sleep, and can assist in reducing anxiety and fatigue. It is likely that you have used lavender in shampoos or soaps. It is mostly added to products to enhance the scent that is capable of taking one to a completely different world. You can purchase the fresh, fragrant flowers and stems of the plant and make the most relaxing tea you can drink to get relief from anxiety and depression. Lavender capsules and oils are also available to take and apply.

Kava kava root

Kava Kava is a plant that is utilized to make a remedy that can help people get relief from anxiety and stress conditions. It is believed to be powerful and has been utilized since the beginning of time for this exact goal. Kava kava can also be utilized to treat sleep-related issues like insomnia. It can help you get peaceful sleep. It's believed to aid in reducing fatigue and assist in reducing anxiety that could have accumulated due to it.

Passionflower

Passionflower is believed to be very beneficial in relieving stress and other stress-related problems. It can help reduce depression and anxiety. It helps to reduce anxiety and helps in boosting confidence. It also helps lower blood pressure and aids to keep you relaxed and in control. Passionflower comes in tablet form and can be purchased through the internet. It is also helpful to reduce irregular heartbeats, and helps in regulating the heartbeats.

Valerian root

Valerian root is very effective in battling mental illnesses. The herb can be utilized to ease anxiety and stress related conditions. It has been utilized in treating asthma due to anxiety. It also helps with hyperventilation. It also assists in the reduction of depression and stress. can aid in boosting the flow of blood to the brain. Valerian root is very effective in helping you to lower stress and attacks of panic. It is available as a tablet and can be purchased on the internet.

Gingko

Gingko is an antiquated Chinese remedy that is employed to treat memory loss and mental problems. Gingko assists in numerous ways, as it affects not only the mind but as well the body. The herb was traditionally utilized to help in the relief from Alzheimer's. It's available as a tablet or powder form and both are able to be taken to alleviate depression and stress. The leaves are are used to make drugs which are made to make the drugs that are used for anxiety and stress. Tablets can be purchased on the internet.

St. John's wort

St. John's wort is one of the most widely used and utilized herbs used to treat anxiety and depression. It has produced remarkable results in people suffering from these mental illnesses and, consequently, is an extremely commonly prescribed natural remedies. The plant is utilized to extract oil which is administered the patients. Hypercin is the chemical which is located in the root, and is believed to have a positive effect in reducing the negative effects of stress on the brain. St. John's wort is offered as a tablet which can be taken in order to relieve these ailments.

Ashwagandha

Ashwagandha is a well-known Indian medicine used to treat mental illnesses. Ashwagandha root and berry are employed for this reason. It is among the most effective herbs you can utilize to treat anxiety disorders. It is often compared to Ginseng that is the Chinese herb that treats anxiety and depression. It is possible to take it in powder or tablet form and get relief from all mental disorders. It is also believed to be beneficial to children since it aids in increasing their concentration and memory. However, it is important to consult the doctor prior to giving this to your children.

It is crucial to speak with your doctor about these medications before you start because some may not be suitable for your body. It is crucial to consult a doctor if you're pregnant or taking any medications.

Chapter 9: In What Ways Do All of These Issues Affect This Generation?

This is a concern that is global and not limited to one country like the US. The disorders, syndromes and mental illnesses are aplenty across the globe. The generation that is growing up with the knowledge that they could be suffering from a mental impairment or at most, an illness that requires treatment.

The younger generation are being diagnosed depression disorders, anxiety disorder, and other disorders that appear daily in children. And that's not even mentioning the anxiety that children already feel due to their parents' anxiety and depression.

Children suffering from anxiety triggered by the anxiety of their parents will be disruptive at school, at home and even in social situations. They are prone to nausea, sleeplessness headaches, stomachaches, and diarrhea and other symptoms, such as irritability, difficulties concentration and fatigue. They are not doing well in the classroom, when they should be performing well.

Parents take their children to the doctor. The doctor tells them they're suffering from X-syndrome or disorder. The doctor then prescribes medication. What can this do? It isn't the solution to this particularly the pharmaceutical ones. They may be better then street drug, however they're nonetheless drugs.

Children create their own strategies to handle situations that bring them sadness and grief. The most effective approach to manage their anxiety in their home environment is to stay clear of the situation altogether or let somebody else handle the issue. They're already feeling anxious, stressed and anxious because of the emotions around them. They are also feeling overwhelmed by the current situation.

This isn't good for them because they'll not be able to cope with the stress later on in life. This can lead to alcohol and substance abuse, even if it's not on the street or prescription medications.

It also results in low self-esteem, low self-confidence and the ability to overlook the things they don't want to be dealing with in their lives. It's much simpler to sip a glass of wine or take a pill and get rid of all the pressures of life.

This is the vision of the near future of all youngsters born in the present. There's nothing to anticipate does it?

A note of note When I was looking into in this publication, I found an informational page that was provided by the National Institute of Mental Health that, in addition, has an official mission statement which reads, "The mission of NIMH is to improve treatment and understanding of mental illness through fundamental or clinical study, and paving the way to prevention treatment, recovery, and treatment." NIMH

There was a post on their website which explains how they intend to assist asfollows "Research to discover brain mechanisms that contribute to anxiety disorders has the potential to identify ways to improve the effectiveness of medications and have less adverse negative effects."

Do you believe "better medicines with fewer adverse consequences" is the solution to the mental disorders of our time? Personally, I believe that they're the root of the mental disorders that affect people including children.

If you're suffering from anxiety or depression, you're unable to move through your day and neither will your children. This is the most significant issue associated with depression and anxiety in the present day. There are different ways to manage it other that are not based on drugs, medications or alcohol.

How to live your Day-to-day Life Even While Dealing with Anxiety

Anxiety can be cured by doing a variety of things that do not involve alcohol or drugs. The research conducted by the author Michel Lucas showed getting more exercising can lower the likelihood of anxiety. Additionally, now that you are aware of how anxiety develops it is possible to work out the adrenaline that is in your body through an exercise, climbing the stairs, or even jumping around in your kitchen to remove the adrenaline from your body.

In a comfortable chair, watching television is sure cause anxiety in your life. Even if you're not thinking about the news, it will still impact your life because it's a part of your brain.

As well, helping your child manage stress is essential for their well-being. As you've seen children are susceptible to anxiety disorders in the early years of their lives. This can hinder them from excelling in school, having social interactions, or in making friends. They are scared, embarrassed and lonely. As they don't know how to deal with the feelings they feel, they turn at substances to ease them get through the day. These substances could be alcohol or drugs, or they might just shut down and watch TV , or play games on their computer or gaming console.

For kids, it's simpler to ignore the issues as opposed to dealing with them, as they aren't aware of what you're experiencing.

They are aware of what it is doing to you and the other person and may suffer from frequent nightmares, make their own imaginary friends, and consume certain food items. Certain aspects of anxiety are normal for children to experience, particularly in the stages. But when parents are overwhelmed with depression or anxiety it causes anxiety, fear and a reluctance to go to certain things and places. This could lead to an anxiety disorder if it is left untreated and impact their daily living.

You can observe the physical signs of anxiety through:

Inability to rest

Unrest

It is difficult to concentrate

Irritability

In school, or at home

The questions they consider include:

Family issues

Peer relationships

Natural disasters

Health

Grades

Performance in sports

Punctuality

The remedy is 10 times. It is essential to talk with your child about the things that are troubling them, and don't just brush it away as normal fears that children have. It's real and terrifying.

There are two kinds of therapy you can employ for helping your child overcome their anxieties before it turns into an issue that will be a problem for them throughout all their lives.

Be aware that there isn't a single method that works for every child. You might need to try various methods to help them respond. Every child is unique and responds to different treatments. Discuss the issue with your doctor to determine the best solution to help them deal with anxiety issues.

Cognitive-Behavioral Therapy

The first is cognitive-behavioral therapy , or CBT. It is a form of therapy that uses talk, and which has, as a matter of fact it has been proven scientifically to be effective in treating anxiety disorders. CBT helps your child learn techniques that can help reduce anxiety. For instance, your child being taught to change negative thoughts with positive ones.

It also teaches them to distinguish unrealistic ideas from reality. The child will apply the lessons they are learning every day. It's a method of helping your child instantly, and they might need it for the rest of their lives. When your child is able to manage their anxiety and stress, you'll notice a dramatic improvement in their personality and temperament.

Medication

The other option is to utilize medication. I'm not a advocate of taking medication, however there are instances that a child has to be calm, so they can put a stop in anxiety. In general, when anxiety has escalated into a disorder, it's the best time to consider taking medication.

There are many that are very effective. These are the categories of medications.

SSR Inhibitors (SSRIs)

They enable your brain to take in more serotonin which is known to enhances mood. They have fewer adverse effects than to tricyclic antidepressants. The medication includes:

Celexa (Generic name Citalopram)

Lexapro (Generic name Escitalopram)

Luvox (Generic name Fluvoxamine)

Luvox CR (Generic name Paroxetine)

Paxil (Generic name Fluoxetine)

Prozac (Generic name Sertraline)

Zoloft

The most frequently reported adverse effects include insomnia and weight gain. These medications are prescribed to those with generalized anxiety disorders and , in larger doses, for obsessive-compulsive disorder or OCD.

Serotonin-Norepinephrine Reuptake Inhibitors (SNRIs)

They perform a double function by increasing levels of the neurotransmitters , serotonin and norepinephrine while also stopping their absorption into the brain cells. Epinephrine and norepinephrine both are hormones produced through the adrenal gland. They form integral to the "flight or fight" response. Norepinephrine (a tension hormone) actually increases heart rate, which means it could be a source of adrenaline. Two of the drugs that are that are used are:

Cymbalta (Generic name Duloxetine)

Desyrel(Generic name: Trazodone)

Effexor(Generic Name: Venlafaxine)

Remeron (Generic name Mirtazapine)

The effects of the medication are stomach upset, insomnia sexual dysfunction, headache and a slight rise of blood pressure. They are often considered to be the initial option for treatment of anxiety disorders.

Benzodiazepines

They are employed for temporary treatment for anxiety. They ease the tension in muscles that is caused by anxiety and tension. They are intended for symptom relief only because they can cause other issues related to dependence (they are addicting).

The drug names for them are:

Clonazepam

Diazepam

Alprazolam

Lorazepam

Tricyclic Antidepressants

These are the most commonly used anti-depressants are the most common. They are highly addictive to the body, and when you stop taking them, it could cause health problems when your body adapts to their own chemical (hormones).

Adapin (Generic term for Doxepin)

Anafranil (Generic name Clomiprimine)

Aventyl (Generic Name: Nortriptyline)

Elavil (Generic name: Amitriptyline)

Luudiomil (Generic Name: Maprotiline)

Norpramin (Generic name Desipramine)

Pamelor (Generic name: Nortriptyline)

Sinequan (Generic term for Doxepin)

Surmontil (Generic name: Trimipramine)

Tofranil (Generic term for Imipramine)

Vivactil (Generic brand name Protriptyline)

While these drugs work however, they can cause a variety of adverse effects, such as the orthostatic hypotension (drop in blood pressure upon standing) urinary retention, constipation, dry mouth and blurred vision.

Always contact your physician if you or your child are experiencing more than the normal adverse symptoms. The abrupt discontinuation of treatment could lead to other health problems.

Chapter 10: Treatment Options for Depression

Alongside the natural remedies discussed mentioned in the previous chapter There are many other options which can aid in helping to reduce the symptoms of depression. This includes:

Relations: While people suffering from depression may show signs of loneliness and desire to remain in a lonely place and feel isolated, relationships can play an vital role as part the treatment. Friends and family can assist tremendously in the process of accelerating your recovery by providing assistance, listening ears or a good companionship, or simply being there to support you. Keep in mind that recovery is not easy to accomplish without support. Patients suffering from depression must engage in activities that involve those who cherish and are concerned about them, even if it's the last thing they would like doing. Being close to those who you care about can serve as a buffer against symptoms increase while also increasing your level of self-confidence and well-being.

Relaxation training: It is often employed to treat symptoms of anxiety. It is essential to realize that depression can be a precursor to anxiety in many instances and that it is possible to reduce depression by simply using relaxation exercises. The training can help relax tight muscles while at the simultaneously reducing behavior and thoughts. Relaxation training can be found in a variety of types, such as progressive muscle relaxation, which allows people to reduce tension and relax certain muscles by voluntary relaxation.

Support groups and forums online Like many other conditions, people suffering from depression can join together to support one another by sharing their personal experiences. They often allow those who have recovered from depressive illness to tell their experiences and share their stories with others suffering from this condition. This can help to show that recovery is possible and is just around the corner. There are forums online, but support groups that meet in person are considered to be more effective.

Sleep and meditation Though people suffering from depression may appear calm at times, the reality is that they have lots going on inside their bodies and minds. Relaxing and sleeping well can be extremely beneficial in relaxing the nerves and mind and you can decrease the negative effects of depression. It is well-known that individuals who suffer from depression may be more susceptible to deterioration of their conditions in the event that they don't rest well. Being able to sleep in a comfortable environment with no interruptions can help enhance your sleep quality and help you unwind. Meditation is also helpful in calming the mind and alleviating depression.

Light therapy with bright light: Light therapy with bright colors has been shown to alleviate the depression-related symptoms. According to a meta-analysis on this treatment, the effects are similar to those found in traditional antidepressants. The therapy is able to be utilized in conjunction with other treatments to maximize outcomes, particularly when employed to treat seasonal depression.

It is important to note that the natural and alternative treatments can be highly effective when combined with other methods of treatment However, they cannot be guaranteed to be as efficient by themselves. Anyone suffering from depression ought to consult with their doctor to determine the best treatment combination. It is usually determined by the degree of the symptoms and signs and also the type of depression can also affect the type of treatment that is used.

Chapter 11: What Different Types Of Depression?

The kinds of depression vary not in relation to the symptoms they present, but rather in the root causes of the issue. According to the conditions that are causing depression there are three major kinds:

Seasonal Depression

It's awe-inspiring to think that many people begin to experience depression around the end of the fall or around the start of winter, particularly in colder climates. This type of depression is sometimes referred to as the 'winter blues', or 'winter depression' or "Seasonal Affective Disorder (SAD)'. In addition, it can be called 'Summer depression or Summertime Sadness' where depression begins with the start of summer. It is more rare.

People who live in an emotionally balanced and healthy state throughout the year begin to feel depressed at the time that summer or winter begin. It's the change in the weather that triggers the beginning of mood swings. People begin to feel completely different after the weather is drastically changed.

Particularly when winter begins and the nights get earlier and people begin to feel exhausted and sluggish. They are not interested in social or work activities and prefer to stay their own company. These mood swings are lessen in intensity and frequency as spring arrives.

Postpartum Depression

Depression following a pregnancy is very common among women. It happens to at least one out of five women following the birth of a child. Depression postpartum - or depression that occurs right after or during the final months of pregnancy - could be serious or mild, dependent on the individual.

Postpartum depression can last weeks or days, and even months in some instances.

New mothers can experience an overwhelming sadness during days which should be most joyful of their life. Depression of this kind will disappear in its own time after a period of time.

Situational Depression

A person who suffers from depression in a situation, as evident from its name, occurs during an event in one's life, such as the loss of a loved one, separation or divorce loss of a job, being unable to complete a course, etc.

This type of depression is actually a result of an extremely stressful period in a person's life. It generally passes over time or after the end of the crisis. However it is possible that therapy might be required.

Premenstrual Depression

A majority of female population in the globe feel sad and depressed throughout their menstrual cycle each month. Within 5 depression is severe to a degree. Women might feel depressed and anxious throughout the day and may become easily annoyed with the people in their vicinity. They may also be unable to focus on their work and are unable to be social with other people.

Manic Depression

The majority of people with manic depression exhibit alternating periods of sadness and happiness. When they feel happy they're extremely active They talk often and fast, take part in numerous things, are sleepy and like to be active all often.

However they can be depressed in other situations and their behavior changes in a flash. They begin to lose interest on their job, preferring the solitude of their home and can get angry.

Apart from these forms of depression, a few sufferers are suffering from atypical depression that is that causes a person to eat a lot and sleep a lot and dysthymia, where an individual may experience an uneasy mood for several months, or even for years; psychotic depression is when the person loses touch with reality and is plagued by depression or delusions, or melancholia when the person who is depressed is prone to react and move slow.

Depression is referred to under a variety of names, particularly among those who aren't aware of its gravity and its consequences, such as the blues, feeling down and under mood, being depressed or melancholia. Depression is a real disease of the mind which can cause a person to feel sad and numb. In the absence of any reason, they feel completely helpless and empty; they could shift completely overnight.

Chapter 12: How to Treat Depression?

The treatment for depression begins when you realize the possibility that you be struggling and need assistance from others. Be assured that there are many effective treatments and natural methods to treat or improve the condition.

You're not alone and you are able to win the battle against depression and gain your happiness back.

You may visit your primary healthcare provider, and they will refer you to an expert who can identify as well as treat the mental illness.

I also suggest that you take someone to be a part of your support system so you don't have any information not missed. Also, you can record the symptoms your experiencing. Also, important personal information, your family's background (if there is any) as well as any medication you may be taking, or medical condition you're experiencing. All of this will aid in the diagnosis process.

You should expect an a thorough interview, physical examination and a lab test. Doctors must determine if there is an underlying medical issue prior to the actual psychological assessment. Don't worry, you're in good hands and the most effective treatment is offered if you are diagnosed.

Following diagnosis, I would recommend that you study all possible about the particular kind of depression you suffer from. You must be prepared for trials and errors to find the right treatment and, once you have found the correct treatment, take it on. Recovery may be rough at times, but you'll reach your goal. Another crucial aspect is that in addition to having a doctor who is supportive on your journey, you should also have social help. It is not necessary to fight this battle on your own. The more you're close to people who are trustworthy or who love you, the greater chance to be able to overcome this challenge.

Here are the treatment options for depression:

Psychotherapy or Talk Therapyis a sure-fire therapy for depressed patients (you must engage and embrace your lessons learned during every session). The sessions will involve an experienced therapist for months, weeks or even years, based on your demands or issues you want to resolve. In the "talk" will provide you with information about the causes of depression, the ability to change your ways of thinking, and also learn new behavior skills that can help you. The majority of the time, it is a blend or combination method of various therapies that are available. The most commonly used approaches are:

Interpersonal therapy focuses is on how you interact with other people and how they impact your. Through this kind of therapy your counselor will be able to modify your habits that are harmful to you.

Cognitive behavioral therapy - the center of attention is your behavior and how you think. In addition, bad habits are identified and eventually altered during the treatment.

Problem-solving therapy - this will focus on specific issues you are facing, and your counselor will assist you in finding specific solutions.

This kind of treatment is advantageous because you are able to continue to apply what you've gained from the treatment when the depression has long gone. It will also allow you to identify the cause of the issue and learn more about yourself and others. It will also help you determine how you think and respond in various situations.

Electroconvulsive therapy as well as other brain stimulation therapies - this kind of therapy has received a negative reputation, however don't worry, it is quite different from the kind of treatment you've seen in horror films. If the psychotherapy or medication treatment failed, electroconvulsive therapy may be able to help people suffering from severe depression. However, it is important to remember that there may be some adverse consequences of this therapy although they aren't usually lasting like memory loss or confusion. The potential benefits as well as side effects will be discussed thoroughly. It is essential to obtain informed consent prior to starting this kind of treatment.

Alternatives/Complementary Treatments:

Apart from the clinically proven treatment options, there's alternative treatments that are natural that you can use or combine with other treatments. However you'll need to consult with your doctor and often it's suitable to mild depressions. Here are some options:

St. John's Wort- This is one of the most sought-after botanical plants throughout the United States that has been utilized for centuries in various traditional and medicinal treatments. The extract of St. John's Wort can be used for mild or moderate depression. However, it is important to remember that it is currently under investigation. Also, you should talk to your physician about it in case it interferes with other medications like birth control pills blood thinners, antidepressants and blood thinners.

St. John's Worth is available in capsules, tables teas, liquid extracts and teas. The daily dose of 900-1200 milligrams is recommended to take between 4 and 12 weeks to observe the positive effects. Also, make sure you buy from reputable suppliers.

Supplements- If you believe that nutritional deficiencies are among the reasons behind your depression, you may want to take a look at a range of supplements you can buy at a pharmacy.

The most popular supplements are Omega-3 fats (should be consumed in an intake of between 2,000 and 4,000 milligrams for improved mood) B-Vitamins (to help stabilize the nerve cell membrane and is vital for maintaining the nervous system), Vitamin D (especially to combat depression during winter) and Valerian (herbal remedy that aids in sleeping and reduce anxiety).

Diindolylmethane DIM DIM uses to treat an enlarged prostate, some cancers, and PMS. Additionally, there are studies that suggest that it's a successful treatment for depressions that result from hormonal imbalance. It also is believed to ease anxiety.

Acupunctureis a technique that is commonly used to treat health issues it involves the use of needles that are finely placed on certain areas of the body. It is increasingly being used for treating depression. There are numerous studies that show positive outcomes when the use of acupuncture, however it isn't yet recognized as a medical treatment. If you are looking to investigate this method ensure that you find an acupuncturist who is licensed and certified.

Alternatives include relaxation techniques, tai-chi yoga, meditation and yoga.

Natural Depression Treatments, in addition to the medications and therapies, or alternatives that you may be exploring, I would recommend that you try other methods of treating depression naturally. What I refer to as natural depression treatments are the modifications you can make in order to alter your attitude and create positive changes in your life.

Here are a few ways to encourage natural depression treatment within your own life:

Establish a routine- depression can be a major cause of confusion, take away the structure of your daily life, and result in confusion or confusion. To combat this begin with simple routines or schedules you are able to adhere to. This will also enable normality to begin to enter your life. As you accomplish your daily check list/schedule/routine, you are also accomplishing mini-goals that will produce regular mini-triumphs that will surely pick up the pieces of your self-esteem.

Eat healthy and nutritious fooditems, specifically ones that are high in Omega-3 fatty acids and Folic acid, which can alleviate depression. Combining healthy eating with regular exercising. Exercise can boost the endorphins in your body and may lead in a more clear and active mind.

Sleeping enough can do wonders for your body and your mind. If you're suffering from depression and have difficulty sleeping, you could be struggling in this regard however, you are able to resolve this (you may seek advice from your therapist on strategies). If, for instance, you're having a difficult sleeping, try changing your routine by sleeping at every night at the same time (develop an routine) or stop watching certain TV series to try to fall asleep Actually it is possible to eliminate all distractions, including television or laptops, smart phones, and many more to help increase your sleep patterns.

Explore something newYou might not be like doing things you once enjoyed However, why not try something completely different? Based on research, experimenting with different things could change the way you think and boost the amount that dopamine is present in the brain (a chemical that can be linked to enjoyment).

Maintain your lifestyleThis may be challenging however, your life should not end because you've been being treated for depression. Make it a point to continue making progress on projects, having a night out with your buddies as well as other activities particularly those recommended by your therapist.

You should have a system of supportIt might be tempting to be a victim and isolate yourself in your sadness, but the truth is that if you're looking to feel better, besides therapy or medication an effective support system will be your lifeline. They could even encourage you to keep fighting the fight.

How can you help a loved One who is Depressed?

Depression isn't just about those who are diagnosed however, it affects those around them, particularly their family members. There are instances when they may feel helpless and helpless, particularly when they feel that they can't assist their loved ones diagnosed with depression. This could cause tension in the relationship, stress, and other negative feelings. The primary thing you need to do is to remain focused on your care and love for your family member or friend.

It is possible that you are not the person who can provide the solution for him or him, yet you could be the one to provide courage, love and support.

Here are a few ways to ways you can assist:

If you suspect that something is going on (if you haven't yet been able to diagnose it) give assistance or an ear to listen. If you are patient, you can get them to talk to you.

Encourage the patient to go to a doctor for treatment and diagnosis.

If you are able, observe or ensure that your loved one adheres to the recommended treatment. Make sure to check in regularly.

Don't dismiss any discussion about suicide. Any comments like this should be addressed to the patient's physician or the therapist. (If you think there's a danger immediately you should not abandon your loved ones or contact 911. You can also call for the National Suicide Prevention Lifeline at 1-800-273-TALK)

Provide the emotional assistance, understanding, and patience that you can offer. If your loved one suffering from depression is causing you to withdraw Do not quit.

Take your loved ones with you to medical appointments.

Engage in new and exciting activities you can both do. This will help free your mind from the problem and may even create bonds between you.

Keep in mind that you cannot "fix" an individual but you can give them the positive energy s/he is in need of. Always remind your loved person that depression is treatable.

I also want to remind you that it's crucial that you don't overlook your personal needs because the presence of a loved one who suffers from depression can also bring you down. Be sure to establish boundaries, or else you could suffer from burnout. It is not your job to be the therapist or caregiver in the end, your loved one has the power to overcome depression. It is also important to carry on in your daily routine or you could be resentful of your family member who is depressed. Also, you require the help you can receive, so share your stress, anxiety and anxieties with your trusted family member or a support group.

When it is identified and properly treated, can be reversed. There are many options that you can discuss with your healthcare professional about the best approach to treat your condition. It is also possible to look into the type of depression you suffer from to gain a better understanding of what you're up against. There are a lot of people who have overcome depression and lead more fulfilling lives following treatment. You too are able to do it! Be able to beat depression by taking one day at a!

Chapter 13: Goal Setting Yourself Goals

We briefly discussed how to accomplish things in the previous chapter, however there's a particular reason for having goals in life. If you're depressed, it's difficult to find motivation to get things done. You don't really desire to. You're so engrossed in your negative thinking patterns that the practical aspects of life don't necessarily register in your mind as something that is important. But they are. The routine you set for yourself determines how far into depression you fall. And when you abandon the routine, you're likely to fall into deeper than you can be able to get out of. So, it is essential to set goals for yourself with the sole purpose of. Goals are designed to see positive results to ensure that the future doesn't appear like a grim future.

Setting goals for yourself

It is only you who can tell the things you don't do. Maybe you aren't keen to lose weight and therefore consume sweets and chocolates for sugar-highs or gain a sense of comfort from what appears to be a miserable life. There are many people who are obese and feel depressed due to having been stuck in a pattern. The reason you make goals is to feel motivated in your daily activities. If you lounge around in your dress gown throughout the day and don't bother to wash, you'll feel like a slob and fall into slovenly routines such as eating out or laying at the television rather than doing activities that aren't just important for your physical health, but are also vital for your mental wellbeing.

It is essential to establish your own routine and include the following aspects:

Cleaning, getting ready and dressing properly

At the table, you can take in fresh ingredients

A walk or some exercise

Social interaction

All night long, you're sleeping

You should drink enough water to meet your body's needs

Be realistic and note down some basic goals you think you'll be able to achieve tomorrow. This could include:

I wash my hair

Showering

Fresh fruit and yogurt to start your day

Drinking an ice-cold glass mid-morning

The dog out for a stroll

Dance to an exercise clip that is shown on TV

It may appear like easy targets, but once you've achieved those goals, it is easy to check the boxes and every time , you celebrate your accomplishment of achieving the goals you set out to do. These may seem like small feats in relation to the overall goal but when you're down, these are goals which aren't easy to achieve even on a low day. When you put your goals in a the form of a list, you can discern clearly when you've completed those tasks. If you manage to get 10/10 completed in a single day, then you're allowed to indulge in something. Make sure to make the desserts healthy, like getting a good bubble bath, enjoying a delicious fruit salad with whip cream or engaging in something you would like to do, like picking a movie to watch with your friends.

Make a point of recollecting all the areas in your life you have to achieve. Social interaction is a crucial one, and it should be a positive, not engaging in the conversation to discuss your depression. Engage in conversation with other people and be kind by listening. If you are constantly talking about depression constantly all you're doing is affirming it. Don't let depression grab a grip on who you are. It is possible that you don't feel the need for engaging in any social activity however in this instance it is a simple message to a friend is going to suffice. It should be about them rather than about you.

If you're not a frequent water drinker be proud of yourself when you are able to sip at least a glass of water. You'll feel good about the food you've cooked for yourself regardless of it being something like a basic salad. Fresh food makes your body feel more energized and drinking plenty of water can alleviate pains and aches. Take your time eating and set an effort to take your time as digestive issues are caused by eating too fast. Set a goal of going into bed by a specific time and turn off all the distracting activities that prevent your from sleeping soundly. Set goals for the day ahead and every of your future ones until you accomplish these things effortlessly, without even worrying about them as they will help you improve your health and keep from falling into depression.

Chapter 14: Evidence Of Depression

There are a lot of things your body and mind are experiencing when you're experiencing depression. These symptoms could include:

Psychological symptoms:

You'll be miserable. The feeling of sadness will last throughout the day and can be different in its intensity. The feelings may be present for weeks, or sometimes even years.

* It may prevent you from having fun in life that you normally would like to do. It takes the enjoyment or excitement out of your daily routines.

* Your thinking process will be slow and inefficient, and your focus is likely to be poor. This can cause difficulty tackling issues, and making decisions and plans.

There are likely to be frequent unsettling thoughts, typically about guilt or that you are a bad or insignificant person. This can result in thoughts of suicide or separating yourself from others because you believe you're not worthy.

The suicidal thought process can lead you to believe that you'd be better off dead , or can trigger feelings of wanting to hurt yourself.

Physical Signs and symptoms:

* You could lose appetite, and suffer from weight loss excessively.

* You may lose the desire to have sexual relations.

You're feeling like you're getting tired even though you're not doing anything physically.

* You're tired however you're unable to rest well, or you are sleep too much. Many suffer from restless and unsatisfying morning wake-ups up to 2 hours earlier than they were scheduled to wake up. You may also be prone to sleeping too long.

* Your speech and activity will be slow.

Any of those symptoms might be a sign that you are being depressed. You must exhibit at minimum five of these signs to be suffering from depression.

What are the main causes of depression?

There is no consensus on the causes of depression. However, it is clear genes play an a significant part in the many instances of depression. Depression is believed to run in families like other mood disorders and about 30% of the predisposition to depression is attributed to genetic factors.

Stressful life events are a factor in the onset or recovery from depression. Conflicts with other people that are ongoing with other people can affect our health, as could other social and environmental stressors like loss of a loved one or something significant, birth or retirement, as well as unemployment. If you're among those who are vulnerable to life's events, these negative ones can be enough to cause or trigger depressive illnesses.

Personality traits of a person could be a major aspect. If someone is depressed, they usually have a negative view towards the world and themselves. They do not appreciate the positive things in life, and the negative issues seem to be overwhelming. Some people are prone to think as this, even when they're not experiencing depression. Also they may have the depressive personality.

The research has revealed that another factor that can cause depression that shouldn't be ignored is medication or physical illnesses. The thyroid hormones, glandular fever influenza, hepatitis, birth medication, anemia, alcohol, and other substances that are abused, as well as other medicines, like those for heart or blood pressure issues may be the cause of the symptoms that are associated with depression.

How to manage depression

The right knowledge about depression is extremely important. The education you receive will give you knowledge that can provide you with a greater degree of control over the disorder. Gaining control can reduce the feeling of despair and improve confidence in yourself and wellbeing. Informing your family about it will also be able to aid them to learn more about your condition and could help you too.

The most crucial piece of advice for anyone who is experiencing a major depressive episode to keep in mind is the fact that depression can be a normal illness and there are many things available that can help. It's also crucial to be aware that depression is a serious illness and is not an indication of character defects or weakness. Recovery is the norm not the exception. The purpose of your treatment is to heal and remain that way. The rate of recurrence in depression is extremely high. Half the people who have suffered from at least one episode of depression will suffer from an occurrence again, and the rates increase as the amount of episodes that have occurred previously. It is important to keep in mind that your family members could be taught to recognize and react in the early symptoms of depression. If treatment is sought out early and appropriately, the extent of the depression may be significantly reduced.

How to deal with depression

The signs of depression can be dealt with so that you be more comfortable. Here are some methods you can aid you in dealing with the symptoms of depression:

BEHAVIOURAL Strategies:

Make goals to be active on a daily basis. You can plan out your days with worthwhile activities by making your own list. This could comprise a checklist of things that you plan to participate in different times through the day. Be sure to adhere to the plan as strictly that you are able to.

What are the kinds of activities you love doing? Make an effort to extend the time that you're engaged in the activities you enjoy.

It is best not to compare your current state of mind or how you are acting now that you're feeling depressed with how you used to be or feel before the time you felt depressed.

You should be sure you reward yourself for your hard work. It is also possible to ask people close to you to encourage and praise you for each small move you take. The process of recovering from depression could be something like learning to walk after injury to your leg.

If you think a task seems too daunting, do not be discouraged. Try breaking it into smaller steps and then begin again slowly.

What should you do if are losing your appetite?

Take less portions of foods you enjoy the most. Do not feel pressured and be patient to finish the meal if dining with friends. It is important to drink lots of water.

What should you do if are losing the desire to have sexual sex

Find things that aren't sexual for you to do with your loved one that you continue to enjoy. Also, you should inform your partner that the loss of desire for affection is a symptom of your depression. Assure them that it isn't an indication of rejection for the other person and that the symptoms will pass over in a short time.

What to do if you're having difficulties sleeping

You should wake up the same time each morning

Do not take napping during the day.

Reduce your tea and coffee consumption if it is excessive (try not to drink greater than 2 or 3 cups per day , and avoid drinking the beverages after 4 pm.

Do not stay awake for longer than 30 minutes. Make yourself up and look for something that is relaxing.

Try exercises that relax you, yoga poses could be an excellent option.

What can you do if your brain isn't functioning properly? thinking or worry

Let the anxiety that you're experiencing to a positive goal. Instead of constantly identifying your concerns, select the ones or two that are significant and then make a the decision to deal with these issues. You could even request a helper from a family member to assist you.

Follow these steps:

Ask yourself what the problem or goal is.

Try listing the possible solutions in five or six in the event that you don't have the same as others do with 3 or 4. Record any thought that pops up to you.

Examine the good and bad aspects of each concept you think of.

Select the most suitable solution that meets your requirements.

Consider the steps you need to take that will be taken to implement your solution

Examine your work when you try to follow the plan. Even if you're not successful be proud of all your efforts.

If you are treated properly, and a thorough understanding of the disorder You can beat depression.

What to do when you're struggling with negative thoughts and are feeling down

The negative thoughts and feelings tend to focus your thoughts on the things you don't enjoy about your life or about yourself. This type of thinking can create a false impression and make your troubles appear more difficult than they actually are.

While focusing on your negative experiences and characteristics that make you depressed it is common to underestimate the strengths of your personality and ways to solve issues. There are many methods you can employ to get an unbiased view of the world.

Make a list of the top three characteristics. You can also seek the help of a family member or family member to highlight these to you. Take the list along with you, and then read it out to yourself every time you are focused on any type of negative thoughts.

Keep a daily record of every little thing you can think of that took place and share these with your loved ones or friends as you meet them.

Remember any memorable events that have occurred in the past. Plan enjoyable occasions for the near future. This can be done through a chat with a companion.

You should consider whether there's another explanation to the unpleasant thoughts about events. Your first thought might be that you're the one to blame. Consider rethinking that idea and record different explanations you could offer for the events you've been thinking about.

Make sure you are engaging in activities that can be beneficial. It is best to avoid spending time doing nothing.

In addition, there are ways to ease the burden of depression. It is important to restore your balance to your brain and also. There has been damage by your brain as a result of long-lasting depression. We will discuss the importance of meditation for your brain, and why you should seriously think about doing it. It's not just "spiritual theological mumbo-jumbo" It's a fantastic technique that's been in use for centuriesand has an excellent reason for it.

Depression is a remarkably complex illness that has an interconnected variety of biological, psychological and sociological causes. However, as we've said before that meditation is among the most effective methods to combat depression.

Chapter 15: The Way to Beat Depression in 8 Steps

One of the largest death-causing factors in recent years is the rising prevalence of depression. It is among the most significant reasons for disability, missing jobs, and broken bonds, etc. It is described as a devastating condition because it takes away the capacity to live a life you enjoy. All the things you familiar with and loved doing every day is now overpowering.

There are several easy steps one can consider as a method of beating depression, as they have been proven to be effective. Depression can be a really uncomfortable feeling, and it's like you're trapped in a dark tunnel without lighting. If there's a chance to overcome the problem, you should consider taking the chance.

Step 1: MINDFULNESS

Mindfulness is recognized as an extremely important practice and method to beat depression. It helps you to be aware of the condition of your body and mind. It is the simplest definition of mindfulness. mindful is the ability to remain conscious of your experiencing. It's all about observation without judgement and being tolerant towards yourself.

When you experience any kind of anxiety or stress Instead of being angry, you take it as a cloud and allow it to disappear into the distance. The entire purpose behind practicing mindfulness is to allow you to spot negative thoughts before they become a burden for you, since it requires a conscious placement of your attention. In mindfulness, you are required to be in a state of constant awareness of the thoughts and bodily sensations, emotions, and the surrounding environment.

It is a state of acceptance in which you pay attention to your thoughts and feelings, without judging them. If one is able to gain an awareness of their own experiences, they are more adept at recognizing their real requirements.

Mindfulness can help us to manage depression by seeing our own self from a distance. Mindfulness can help you react to situations in a relaxed manner that does not affect your heart, mind or body. It can improve the overall quality of life because it helps us develop the ability to see, understand and be clear. Being able to watch the thoughts that flow through your head will enable you to slowly ease your struggles to deal with this.

It is , therefore, one of the most crucial actions to take in order to conquer depression because it can help you manage all the elements which contribute to depression e.g. negative thoughts, anxiety, pain etc.

STEP TWO 2: Physical Exercise

Exercise is one of the most important practices that people incorporate into their daily routines to improve their overall health. According to research, depression-related symptoms are often alleviated by working out. For those suffering from depression, it is often it difficult to incorporate exercise an integral part of their daily routine since it's always the last thing on their minds. What they aren't aware of is the significant difference exercise can bring.

Exercise does more than just act on depression, but it has been proven that it can help in preventing and improving a range of health issues e.g. high blood pressure, diabetes etc. It boosts your mood making you feel better and removing the signs and symptoms of depression.

What exercise can do to decrease depression is the release of happy brain chemicals. It also reduces the inflammation-related chemicals in the immune system that could make depression worse and also raises body temperature, which creates an calming effect. This increases confidence and takes their minds off of anxiety.

A lot of people think of exercise as simply attending the gym or performing all those boring exercises, however exercise can involve various activities, many of which aren't requiring much effort. It could be as simple as taking care of your garden or washing your car, or simply strolling around the block so long as it keeps you off of your couch or bed and keeps you active.

Many doctors recommend exercising to nearly all of their patients because the positive effects of exercise are usually felt instantly. A lot of people who suffer from depression constantly feel as if they're out of the control of their life. exercising can help them gain back control over their bodies, which can lead to healing.

It is important to keep in mind that any form of exercise is effective so the exercise is appropriate for you and you perform enough of it. Whatever your age, weight or color exercising regularly can help you live more healthy and happy life.

Step 3: GETTING ENOUGH SLEEP

Sleep deprivation is a problem that's common that can affect your mood, energy levels and health, as well as your capacity to function. Although overcoming depression isn't effortless or simple but it's not impossible. And getting sufficient sleep is one measure you must do to beat it.

The process of getting better can take time however, you can achieve happiness by making the right decisions and taking the right actions every day. Depression can cause sleep changes and you could be sleeping insufficiently or you're sleeping too often. In all, your mood is affected and in order to manage depression, you need to have a more restful sleeping schedule and develop healthy habits of sleeping.

It's not that difficult to keep a healthy sleep habit , as with just some willpower and a simple change to your routine, you'll be able to achieve it. Sleep is essential to boost your energy levels, and having too much of it, or even too little, can significantly affect your mood and mood.

Depression isn't something you should ignore as it's a serious illness that impacts your consume food, sleep, and think. There is a link between depression and sleep, in that depression can trigger sleep issues and problems with sleep could exacerbate depression problems. People who suffer from insomnia are at greater chance of developing depression opposed to those who rest well.

To get the best sleep, it is important to maintain an established routine for sleeping by getting up at every day at the same hour and waking up at in the same hour. It is not recommended to watch television at night, however you should engage in relaxing and quiet pursuits like reading or relaxing in a warm bath. Also, one should not be working late and stay away from the use of caffeine.

Sleep is essential and the appropriate quantity of it is suggested. How you sleeping affects how you live your day, mental vigor, productivity as well as your emotional health. Therefore, it is essential to rest for 7-9 hours each evening.

STEP FOUR: SUNLIGHT DISPOSURE

The daily exposure to sunshine assists to keep your internal clock on. This assists in regulating the cycle of sleep and wake, that allows us to get an enjoyable night's rest and improves our mental and physical health. The lack of exposure to sunlight increases depression as well as reducing our energy levels which are crucial to maintain our health as it helps us perform our daily tasks.

If you're exposed to sunlight, your body naturally produces an increase in certain vitamins, which result in a decrease in certain depression-related symptoms. To increase the efficiency of the process you can incorporate exercise into the time they're getting sunlight e.g. walking. It is mandatory to take 30 minutes of sun each day.

The sun's rays not only boost your mood but also raises the levels of an antidepressant that is natural that is present in the brain. According to studies the brain produces more of the chemical responsible for boosting mood (serotonin) during sunny days as opposed to dark days. Insufficient sunlight and lower levels of serotonin can trigger the appearance of the seasonal anxiety disorder (SAD) and is the reason that its symptoms are typically felt in winter.

Most people, regardless of regardless of whether they suffer with depression, or are not feel at ease when the sun is out. To enjoy the sunshine, you must open your eyes and avoid wearing sunglasses as when the bright light hits the retina, it triggers the optic nerve that sends an impulse to the region of the brain that controls creation of serotonin and Melatonin.

Step Five: Omega-3 Fat ACID

Research has proven the omega-3 fatty acids can be highly effective in the treatment of moderate to mild depression. Fish oil is believed to be a potent supply of Omega-3 fats, which have been proven to play an important and vital role in brain functioning. According to medical professionals that suffer from depression are thought to have low levels of neurochemicals EPA and DHA which are derived through omega-3 acids.

If you're interested in taking omega-3 fats supplements, they aren't the only option. One could also eat fish once or twice during the course of the week, which is the most effective way to supply your body with adequate omega-3 fatty acids. Omega-3 Fatty acids are vital nutrients, which means that the body isn't able to produce them, so they must be sourced from food. In addition to fishing, you can get it from nuts and seeds.

Antidepressant medications have recently continued to cause concern about their negative effects. This is why eating large amounts of Omega-3-fatty acids is recommended since it provides a powerful shield against depression. It is crucial for a healthy central nervous system, which is responsible for the transmission of signals from the eyes to the brain, and to ensure heart health.

STEP SIX SOCIALIZATION

People who suffer with depression are prone to separating themselves from their peers but do not realize that it's through our antisocial behaviours that we increase feelings of loneliness, hopelessness and despair. It is recommended to go out and meet with family and friends because they are the ones who can help you to come to awareness of the value of living by giving the meaning of life.

Socialization is the best way to build relationships with others and create feelings of hope and appreciation. Humans are social creatures and by socializing while maintaining an impression being connected to others, it assists in reducing stress. Socializing can be described as online chat as well as spending time with friends and family members calling as well as joining clubs. These are just some of the things that can create a sense of security, safety as well as belonging and pleasure.

STEP 7 Step 7: READING

Many doctors have spoken about why reading is important as a method of coping with depression. Reading can help combat depression as the pleasure of reading books brings great relief that can be a sign that someone is finally waking from their plight and escaping from the dark clouds which never seemed to go away.

There's always a good book that will provide a different perspective on life for everyone. It's not just about the book, but rather how it does to you. A lot of books can be a way to enhancing your positive outlook which is the reason it's via positive thinking that we can recover. By reading, one is able to free their mind from stress.

If you establish reading as a regular part of your life, you will see that your mind develops new interests instead of being focused on negative thoughts. The most effective way to alter your mood is by changing the way you think. Make books your instrument in changing your thoughts, and in turn decreasing depression.

STEP 8 A : GOD BLESSING

In the words of a famous quote, "holding on to anger is as if you drink poison and expect somebody else to be killed." If we keep grudges, we are the only ones who feel the anger, and we're the only ones taking in from the inside. Whatever happened to you, don't let the hurt to define you because it affects only you, not them. Find a space within your heart to accept forgiveness.

Forgiveness isn't just about being kind to others, but also about forgiving yourself and situations. Don't blame yourself for the mishaps you have experienced and don't put blame on situations. Everything happens for reasons and at times when you feel overwhelmed, you need to learn that there's always hope at the end of the tunnel.

Keep your thoughts and emotions in check and you'll be able to beat depression of any kind. When you're able to let go and forgive, you can feel more content and provide your mind with energizing thoughts that will be able to conquer depression.

Chapter 16: Living With Depression

Implementing permanent lifestyle changes into your day-to-day activities is the most simple and effective method to fight anxiety and depression. Beyond taking antidepressants, or attending meetings with psychiatrists inner reflection and the desire to improve one's outlook on life is the main element for treating depression. Implementing a healthy lifestyle can reduce the likelihood of suffering from depression again.

Below is a listing of lifestyle changes that can be beneficial if implemented regularly:

Exercise

Studies have proven it is possible to establish a substantial link with exercise, depression and. Individuals who exercise regularly or engage in regular physical activity tend to have a more positive mood and lower risk of developing depression when compared with those who don't.

When you exercise, your body releases endorphins which cause a feeling of feeling of euphoria. This is known as the "runner's elevated". Endorphins create a more stimulating and positive method of processing information. Additionally, they act as an analgesic that helps to reduce the perception of pain. They work similar to morphine. However, in contrast to morphine, endorphins released by the body won't result in dependency or dependence.

There is no need to be a rigorous training regimen for the upcoming basketball event to be able to notice the impact. Just a half hour walk can have a huge impact. If you're looking to maximize the benefits of exercising it is recommended to take part in physical activities for at minimum an hour each day.

A regular exercise routine has shown to help improve and maintain sleep patterns, decrease stress and improve self-esteem. It also helps combat anxiety and depression. Additionally, it has many other benefits which include: strengthening your cardiovascular system reduces blood pressure, improves bone strength and reduces body fat and increases muscle strength.

Exercise in any form can ease depression symptoms. But, due to safety concerns medical professionals and experts generally suggest moderate exercise such as gardening, biking, chores at home, dancing golf, jogging swimming, walking, tennis/badminton, yard work and even meditation (such like yoga). If you are deciding on the kind of exercise you wish to do, you must to first ask yourself what type of physical exercise am I most comfortable with? Do I prefer solo or group-based activities? What kind of exercise routines best suit my needs? Have I physical constraints that hinder my options? Do I have a specific purpose in mind (For instance, gaining strength of muscles or weight loss)?

Be sure to follow the sun!

Studies have shown research has shown that Vitamin D has the potential to reduce depression symptoms. Wear an adequate amounts of sunscreen to ensure that you don't cause skin burns. Only spend a few minutes outside.

Keep an eye on your thoughts

You must make a conscious effort to monitor the way you think or the way you think about the world within you. Your pessimistic and negative inner voice may be fueling your depression. Be aware of your inner conversation with yourself. How do you respond to events, situations and emotions? How do you relate to other people?

Nutrition

The right type and quantity of food is crucial not just for your physical health, but also your mental health. When you make sure you eat balanced and healthy meals throughout the day, you'll reduce your mood swings and maintain your energy levels.

Do the things that will bring you happiness

Based on a study carried out by the National Institute of Health, dropping interest in things you once enjoyed is a sign of clinical depression. Although it may seem like you're no longer enjoying your hobbies or social event, this can help you overcome depression. Don't let depression define you. Don't let it ruin your relationship with people.

Social Support

When you're feeling down when you are depressed, you may block out people. It is easy to become isolated from the world. That's one of the worst things you can do. Feelings of despair and despair is only aggravated by feeling isolated. There is no one who is completely isolated. You'll need every bit of help you can receive from your family and friends. Stay in contact with your loved ones and friends. If you'd like to, you can join a support or class community for those suffering from depression.

If you can, try to be able to meet in person with others. According to research carried out at Leeds University in the United Kingdom those who spend much time talking online , sending emails and text messages, instead of meeting face-to-face are more susceptible to anxiety and depression than those who don't. That's why individual interaction is the key. Don't depend on technology. If you'd like to communicate with someone and talk to them in person. Making a visit to a family member intimately can not only make your reunion more memorable, but also make it more personal.

Sleep

Studies have shown that sleep can have a profound effect on mood. If you're not getting enough rest, the signs of depression can become more severe. If you're not sleeping you are likely to become depressed, moody, tired and easily annoyed. This is why it's vital to get enough rest each night. You should sleep for at least 8 hours a day.

Avoid Chemicals!

Whatever the tempting appeal may be, you should not ever give in to the short-term relief offered by fats alcohol, sugar and other substances. These substances only make you feel more miserable about your self. Keep in mind that a problem could not be resolved by a different issue. Take the lead. Avoid a temptation like alcohol, drugs, or nicotine.

Find your purpose

Whatever cliché it may sound, you have to identify your goal in life so that you remain motivated to continue living your life. Research has proven that people with a strong sense the purpose of their lives are more likely to face all the challenges and ups and downs of life. A sense of purpose can serve as a sort of psychological shield against all the challenges one might face in a particularly challenging day. The key to passion is the need to have a purpose. If you're looking to live every day with energy and enthusiasm and determination, then you must find your passion in life. Consider Gandhi and Nelson Mandela. They were faced with a myriad of trials and struggles and even despair, but they were motivated, that ignited their passion and inspired their determination.

Don't get too hard on yourself!

Be sure to be gentle with yourself. Don't be too smug about skipping a workout or similar. It is important to realize that making long-term lifestyle changes during depression isn't an easy feat. Do not overburden yourself with unrealistic goals. Begin by taking small steps at a. There's no need to hurry. You have plenty of time to spare. Think of it as an endurance race rather than a sprint, and be grateful for the journey, and for yourself as you go along.

Discover yourself as you go along Find yourself, dive deep and conduct a soul search as long as you can. Beginning at the beginning and throughout the way, you must love yourself. The good as well as the bad, the short-comings and everything else, because love for yourself is the most important factor to overcome depression.

Chapter 17: How Can You Do? do about it?

Breathing is known as a programmable capability of the body, which is controlled through the respiratory framework and controlled via the central nervous system. Breathing is an action of the body when confronted with pressure, and there is an abrupt change in rate and tempo of breathing.

This is a part of our body's "fight or Flight" system , and is part of the body's response to stressful situations. It is possible for people to regulate their breathing and studies have shown that when we are able to regulate our breathing patterns, we are able to manage pressure and other health-related conditions like anxiety and depression.

Controlled breathing, when used in yoga, tai-chi, and other reflective exercises can also be utilized to attain a state of unwinding. Breathing techniques that are controlled can lessen the related situations:

* Anxiety problems

* Panic attacks

* Chronic fatigue disorder

* Asthma assaults

* Acute suffering

* High Puls

* Insomnia

* Stress

Breathing and Stress

The main function that breathing has is transport oxygen into the body , and remove carbon dioxide out of the body via the lung. The muscles around the lungs, like the stomach, regulate the movement of the lungs just like the muscles located within the ribs.

A person who is under stress changes their breathing patterns. In general, when you're in a state of anxiety, you take smaller, less shallow breathing with the help the shoulder muscles rather than the muscles of your stomach to regulate your breathing in the lung.

This type of breathing can intrude on the gas-to-gas ratio of the body. Hyperventilation, or a shallow breathing pattern can draw out the sensation of anxiety, as it causes the effects of anxiety to increase.

Breath Relaxation Response

In the event that you feel unfocused or uneasy, relax the body and breathe slowly and gently through your nose to assist in evening out the rhythm of your breathing. The breathing technique of a person who is relaxed can help calm the body's sensory system that handles the automatic components of the body.

The controlled breathing process can also alter the physical condition of an person, for example decreasing the heart rate, reducing stress hormones, reducing the development of lactic corrosive muscles' tissues as well as regulating carbon dioxide and oxygen levels within circulation.

Sympathetic and Parasympathetic Nervous System

Instances of deep breathing stimulate your Parasympathetic nervous system also known as the PNS which is in charge of bodily exercise in a relaxed out state, or when you are in a solitary state. However hyperventilation is a powerful force that supports the opposite.

It is believed that the Sympathetic Nervous System also known as SNS is the one in charge of physical activities that trigger the response of fight or flight that occurs in the body when stress is detected. The SNS can be viewed in two frameworks as follows: PNS is the quiet one that is quiet, while SNS is the crazy and unthinking sister who is always close to mental breakdown.

In terms of the components of our bodies that we control, one of the most important that we have control over is our breathing. It is the method by which we can rehabilitate our bodies. When you alter how you breath, you will assist different parts of your body function regularly to avoid the real reaction to stressors.

Breathing Exercises to Reduce Anxiety

There are three breathing exercises which you can try to help you overcome anxiety and depression. As we have mentioned the process of hyperventilating may greatly intensify anxiety and stress. Relaxation exercises are a great way to help you reduce the negative effects of stress and anxiety.

Coherent Breathing

The controlled breathing exercise allows you to decrease your breathing rate dramatically and increases the heart rate variability, or on the other hand , HRV which is a part of the Parasympathetic Nervous Systems.

The technique is easy and is a breeze to do anywhere. Start by taking a full breath in, then counting to five. After you count back to five while you exhale. The technique requires you to breathe at a pace of five breaths every minute.

Watch how the changes in your breathing affect the HRV that is responsible of switching your sensory structure from the PNS into the SNS or the reverse. What it boils down to is that a higher HRV means the cardiovascular system is more efficient and a more grounded response to stresses.

Resistance Breathing

Respiratory breathing, like its name implies it is breathing in a way that causes resistance during the movement of air throughout the body. It's a method to breathe that restricts the airway or utilize objects like a straw that allows breathing in and out occurs. An easier way to accomplish this is to inhale using your nose rather than your mouth.

Another method of practicing breathing resistance is to relax during recitation or singing. This is a feasible method to accomplish this because the vocal cords are thin along the air's pathways.

Breath movement

Breath movement is the process where you think of breathing. It makes you inhale as if you're driving oxygen towards the top of your head. This is followed by eliminating all carbon dioxide in your body. While doing this, you must imagine that you are taking your breath away from your lungs to the top level of your head.

Learning to control your breathing will drastically reduce the effects of pressure and assist you overcome your anxiety disorder. Utilizing breathing techniques that are controlled like the ones mentioned above, along using mindfulness, will ensure that your mind is calm and at the same time, focused on the present.

What Can You Do to Manage Your Thought to manage anxiety

In the event that you frequently experience bizarre and bizarre thoughts that get you frustrated and you want to clear these thoughts out of your mind If so, you'll be happy to know that you're able to accomplish that by learning the most efficient method to handle your thoughts to help you manage your stress levels.

Although it's not uncommon to experience bizarre and strange thoughts from time to time However, what makes them less uncommon and unusual is when they repeat and when you are having difficulties in ignoring the occurrences.

These thoughts that are irrational can create dread due to the how the idea is so irritating in its nature. In the event that you have to make the possibility of dealing with your concerns, you'll need to understand the factors about those thoughts and their bases, and the best way to stay away from them.

Manage Your Anxiety by Controlling Your Thoughts

If you're having trouble calming your mind with insane thoughts, it is because you are experiencing anxiety-related thoughts. Anyone who isn't experiencing the negative effects of anxiety is likely to have difficulty understanding the many ways anxiety affects your body as well as the mind.

The real reason behind this is that people experience anxiety at different times in their lives. A few common scenarios that create anxiety include the job interview, a testing, or even having someone ask you out.

In any case this, these instances of anxiety typically disappear following the end of the event. However, people who suffer from anxiety disorders differ from the normal anxiety that others experience.

Anxiety disorders may be a source of stress for both the emotional and physical aspects of our lives that can result in a significant disparity. The creation of crazy and frightening thoughts is just one of the primary negative effects that people suffering from anxiety face and manage.

Anxiety can alter one's perceptions and cause you to think and acknowledge that you're getting lost in the world around you. It can make you believe that you're losing your mind, and by doing this, are getting insane.

If you're suffering from these adverse effects You don't need to worry about it, in addition, they're simply the results of your anxiety-related thoughts.

What is the best way to let anxious Thoughts Start?

There are distinct anxiety-related thoughts that could be thought to be insane. The thoughts that arise are usually rooted in anxiety, but the majority originate from the anxiety symptoms you could suffer from.

Undesirable Images

The people who suffer from the negative effects of obsessive-compulsive disorder OCD are the ones who frequently experience images of a negative nature. The images that are undesirable are usually associated with their feelings of worry, anxiety and the need to protect their own lives as well as the lives of those they love.

Every now and then, these dreadful images may be triggered by the thing they fear the most. For instance, people who suffer from the negative affects of OCD might imagine some kind of severe brutality, which could be extremely distressing. Due to this discomfort they will have to shut the majority of doors.

On contrary they might be imagining the possibility of a massive fire to happen, therefore they regularly look to determine if gas is flowing. This is a legitimate connection to their fear.

Unwarranted Fears

The root of worry is anxiety. In this way, someone experiencing anxiety is subject to strange stressors that often seem excessive. This makes them fear about the possibility of something catastrophic happening. The stress-inducing effects is often incredibly pervasive and subjective. Be whatever it is the outcome is the sufferer of anxiety feeling an odd feeling, which can make them feel uncomfortable.

The Fear of losing your mind

The real fear that anxious sufferers are going insane stems due to the effects of anxiety that are too intense that they might think they're insane and losing the battle. The specific feeling of anxiety can turn your head through a myriad of irritants and rapid thoughts that can be extremely difficult to manage.

This anxiety can be unreasonable enough that it can affect everyday activities and may greatly affect the lives of people with anxiety disorders.

The most effective method to Prevent Anxious Thoughts

The anxiety you experience is affected by your thoughts and the way you think is dependent on anxiety. If one thing is compounded by the other, the situation may become extremely difficult to manage. Here are some methods to help you to keep a distance from worrying and break the cycle of anxiety.

Check out the Thought for what it is.

It is preferential not to think about the particular notion because of the fear that goes with the thought. Whatever the crazy thought may be when you are able to face it, your thoughts will never again cause you to avoid the thought. It does not matter when that specific idea comes up.

Think of the idea you want to create.

Another method to tackle your thoughts is to create the thoughts before they ever occur. When your brain has become accustomed to thinking about it, your fear will be crushed.

The Thoughts you have on Paper

One method that professionals use to help people who are anxious manage their anxiety is to document the troubling thoughts as a way to clear it from the mind. If someone is having trouble focusing writing them down on paper is similar to putting them somewhere where they are able to remain forever and allow the brain to loosen and not have to be concerned about it again.

The routine of recording frightening and agitated thoughts is a way to soothe the mind and allows it to ignore these thoughts in the longer term. These are just a few of the easy methods you can begin to implement to control anxious thoughts that pop up randomly. Although you'll, in any event, need to deal with your primary anxiety These simple steps will help you to stop mind-numbing thoughts in their lines.

Chapter 18: The Way to cultivate a positive attitude even when you're depressed

In the preceding chapter, we spoke about positivity as the antithesis of negativity. This is the main catalyst that ignites the fire of depression. We also discussed an overall approach to creating a positive attitude within us. We'll speak about specific strategies to help you develop a positive outlook even when suffering from depression.

Give Thanks

One of the most important virtues of life is gratitude and can assist people to be less angry, less discontented, less jealous as well as less jealous, less critical, less sad and happier and more hopeful. The foundation of gratitude is gratitude. on which positive energy is built. Therefore, the first step to being able to beat negative thoughts - and in turn depression is to be thankful for all the blessings we enjoy and the people around us with affection, and other positive things.

The process of developing or cultivating a thankful attitude in your life can be achieved in various methods, however for me personally, one of the most simple and most effective methods to do this is through journaling. Journaling is a great way to develop a heart of gratitude by writing every thing you're thankful for and are grateful of on a sheet newspaper or inside your own notebooks as an integral part of your morning routine. It doesn't matter whether the majority of the items you write every day are items you've been grateful for over the past several weeks or days. It's important to keep being reminded by your daily list of the things you're thankful for and are grateful for. As you keep reminding yourself of these things and the more you will realize that life isn't all that awful and that there are less reasons to be sad.

Check out the Side that is Bright Side

William James, the author of one of the most popular self-help books ever written, Acres of Diamonds stated that as a person (or woman or both, depending on what the situation may be) thinks, so is the case with him (or the woman). Mahatma Gandhi believed that your thoughts will become your actions, words and ultimately your destiny. It is therefore essential to keep your mind in the right direction and focus on the positive aspects in your life, or in your circumstances.

You might say that it's not as simple as it seems! Well, you're right. However, it doesn't mean that it's not possible or even feasible. One thing is that I have never advocated denying the awful events that are happening throughout your day. What I'm asking for you to think about is consider them less and focus more on what's feasible. In doing this you prepare your mind to find solutions and for joy instead of insurmountable issues and despair.

One way to build the practice of looking at the positive aspects of life is by taking your negative thoughts out of the way. What exactly do I mean by this? Begin by becoming mindful or alert when negative thoughts dominate your thoughts or you are able to make negative remarks. When you notice yourself thinking or talking negative thoughts, don't get down on yourself or blame yourself for doing it. Instead, acknowledge in a non-judgmental manner that you have did or said such negative thoughts or statements. Then, continue by telling yourself at minimum two positive thoughts about the circumstances or situation which led you to speak or think negative thoughts or words. In doing this you will outnumber or crush your negative thoughts by replacing them with positive ones.

You may, for instance, have encountered an accident when you were driving to work. The possibility of getting an additional yellow ticket for tardiness this week prompted you to say or think that it was going to be a bad working day for you on the third consecutive day this week. If you come to the realization of these thoughts or phrases, accept it as a fact and admit the fact that you made the decision to say or think about it, but as soon as you can consider at least two things you are thankful for, for instance, the reality that you're taking your own car to get there. This means that you can get a car for yourself and travel in comfort and also you're employed in a position that allows you to afford the luxury of a car and other similar things.

There are other things you can do to make it simpler and less personal for you, but it will require some courage. Have someone you trust be accountable to you and tell that you've slipped back to the negative zone, so that you can fill in the gaps that you aren't conscious of. But, one of the most difficult aspects to this is that it could result in anger or depression. This could happen if those who you'll request to take care of it are inclined to use the most unhelpful manner of speech.

There's a way around for this. You can negotiate with that person to allow the other person to use an appropriate cue phrase that is preferably humorous when they spot you falling back into negativity without knowing. In this way you reduce the chance of using a loud voice or apparent rude word of encouragement and, consequently, reduce the chance of your depression or anger being provoked. When you're reminded of it, consider at least two positive things about the circumstance or situation that you're currently in.

Leave Things Behind

Depression is like an individual in the sense that it can possess the ability to think on its own occasionally. There are occasions when it brings to mind things that are depressing that happened in the past, such as when the school bully threw your underwear's garter that far up your back that it turned into a hoodie before all students that resulted in a lot of laughter and jeers. Depression can hold the weight of your negative experiences of the past, resulting in a heavy emotional burden that can make the condition more difficult to overcome.

If depression causes the same to you, how is the best way to end this dependence on your extremely negative past or reduce its power within your own life? One of the most effective and most efficient methods is to practice meditation. The basic idea behind the practice is to improve your mind's capacity to see your negative experiences as gone and unimportant and will allow you to let them go from your life. Here's how you can do it:

If you are able to recall some negative incident in your past, that you'd like to forget, shut your eyes (assuming it's appropriate to do so) and take your breath deeply, and then repeat "gone" while you exhale, then you can open your eyes.

- Now you must accept that the negative thought, all discomforts that it may cause and any annoyances of the past have gone from being a part of the present to one of never again, i.e., extinction.

Refrain from the fact that what is past isn't able to control your life from now on. The present is yours and your past negative - including the thoughts and feelings that go with it - will have no influence on your life.

It's that easy and simple. But here's the part that can be a bit difficult it'll feel like nothing is happening for the first fifty or hundred times. You may think that you're thinking about these things. Keep on your toes that brain is similar to your physical muscles, in that it is able to be taught to remember things and strengthen through consistency and persistence. By continuing to practice this leaving-things-behind technique even if it doesn't seem to be "working" at first, it will bear fruit at the right time. There's nothing to lose since it's not something that takes much effort or time or money but the rewards could be life-changing.

Change Your Lenses

This isn't referring to your eyeglasses , but to the mental lenses through which you view your world, and how you interpret your experiences and events. As an example instead of deciding to view a failed attempt to make something happen to be a loss, take a look towards it through the point of view that it's yet another attempt at learning about what isn't working, which will lead you closer to figuring out what can be achieved through elimination. Thomas Edison thought this way by observing the countless "failed" lighting bulb experiments until he found the right solution!

For instance instead of complaining about the fact that you're eating the leftover turkey you ate the previous night's dinner consider it as being blessed to be able to enjoy turkey for two days when most people are unable to afford it only once in a year! Another example is instead wondering why you're not making your goal income then consider what you could accomplish that goal! Reframe your thoughts and questions to positive ones and allowing your brain to be trained to think about the positive outcomes that can be brought to fruition rather than thinking about the less positive possibilities.

Visualize

There's a good reason behind the claim"pictures paint thousand words. It is! Why is that? The human brain is wired to think through pictures and hence the name photographic memory. If you establish the habit of daily visualizing specifically about your dreams, hopes and goals and goals, you're essentially informing your mind's subconscious to pursue it, increasing your chances of being successful. The more successful you are your life, the less stressed you'll feel in your life!

Even if the things you're picturing aren't yet manifesting by imagining in your head the things you want to accomplish or are planning to achieve in the near future will help you become positive and optimistic about these things. Hope is among the most effective antidepressants as hopelessness is among depression's main characteristics. The more precise you visualize, the better you will be able to motivate yourself to manage your depression better. Keep in mind, hope delayed is hope denied. By creating visualizations of your goals your routine, you will not put off hope.

Get rid of the Balance

One of the most common reasons why people feel depressed is a strong sense of feeling "not sufficient." The issue in"not enough "sense" can be that, most of the times, it's incorrect. One of the primary causes of many people's perception of feeling "not adequate" is the notion of being "well-balanced," which means having a good record in every area of life. This belief system affirms "Never think that someone is at the top in his profession and is lavishly rewarded in terms of power, fortune and fame. They must have to be "well-rounded."

If you've have read Cal Newport's bestseller Deep Work, you'll realize that living the perfect lifestyle all the time is not the ideal method to live your life. It's because you won't capable of maximizing your gifts and talents due to being driven by the "need" to compensate for your weaknesses which may not be of any importance to you in the first place. Let that be known you're Bill Gates. It's obvious that he's not proficient in the area of finance, but because he poured all of his effort into making the most of his gift or power that is programming computers which is computer programming, he managed to earn enough money that he's now able to employ the top accounting professionals and finance managers around the globe to oversee his company's finances! He's gotten rid of the balance to concentrate on his strengths and simply employed or asked for help to perform the tasks the area he's not a specialist in.

If you are focused on your strengths and talents You'll increase your odds of success in the things that matter most to you. If you're successful and grow, the more you'll see that you're far from a hopeless or worthless individual and you've got something worthwhile to contribute towards the greater good of humanity. One who is aware of his worth and is able to maximize his strengths and talents is unlikely to be depressed or remain there.

Conclusion

I hope this book is helpful in getting you started feeling confident about yourself and your life. Rememberthat depression is serving as a wake-up signal to honor yourself, recognizing your feelings and growing in exciting, new ways. I have witnessed a lot of people overcome depression and be grateful for the time they endured it as it made them stronger and wiser. They also became more compassionate. I'm confident that you'll be among them. You can do it!

It is the next thing to do: act using any of the methods I've outlined previously. I am aware that depression can stop people from feeling motivated to take action however, I guarantee you that if you follow any of the suggestions mentioned above and you'll instantly be feeling relief. Actually, you might be smiling at how great you feel now.

www.ingramcontent.com/pod-product-compliance
Lightning Source LLC
Chambersburg PA
CBHW070100120526
44589CB00033B/1098